eau Official Organ of the European Association of Urology

# European Urology

AF885292



KARGER

Printed in Switzerland
on acid-free paper by
Druckerei Schüler AG, Biel

Appears 6-weekly;
2 volumes per year (8 issues)

European Urology

**Submission:** Only original papers written in English are considered and should be sent to:

Prof. C.C. Schulman
Department of Urology
Hôpital Erasme
Cliniques Universitaires de Bruxelles
Route de Lennik 808
B-1070 Brussels (Belgium)

Manuscripts should be submitted in *triplicate* (with three sets of illustrations of which one is an original), typewritten double-spaced on one side of the paper, with a wide margin.

**Conditions:** All manuscripts are subject to editorial review. Manuscripts are received with the explicit understanding that they are not under simultaneous consideration by any other publication. Submission of an article for publication implies the transfer of the copyright from the author to the publisher upon acceptance. Accepted papers become the permanent property of 'European Urology' and may not be reproduced by any means, in whole or in part, without the written consent of the publisher. It is the author's responsibility to obtain permission to reproduce illustrations, tables, etc. from other publications.

**Arrangement**

*Title page:* The first page of each paper should indicate the title (main title underlined), the authors' names, and the institute where the work was conducted. A short title for use as running head as well as the full address of the author to whom correspondence should be sent are also required.

*Full address:* The exact postal address complete with postal code must be given at the bottom of the title page. Please also supply Phone and Fax numbers.

*Key words:* For indexing purposes, a list of 3-10 key words in English is essential.

*Abstract:* Each paper needs an abstract of up to 10 lines.

*Small type:* Paragraphs which can or must be set in smaller type (case histories, test methods, etc.) should be indicated with a 'p' (petit) in the margin on the left-hand side.

*Footnotes:* Avoid footnotes. When essential, they are numbered consecutively and typed at the foot of the appropriate page.

*Tables and illustrations:* Tables and illustrations (both numbered in Arabic numerals) should be prepared on separate sheets. Tables require a heading and figures a legend, also prepared on a separate sheet. For the reproduction of illustrations, only good drawings and original photographs can be accepted; negatives or photocopies cannot be used. When possible, group several illustrations on one block for reproduction (max. size 181 × 223 mm) or provide crop marks. On the back of each illustration, indicate its number, the author's name, and 'top'. Color illustrations are reproduced at the author's expense.

*References:* In the text identify references by Arabic numerals [in square brackets]. Material submitted for publication but not yet accepted should be noted as 'unpublished data' and not be included in the reference list. The list of references should include only those publications which are cited in the text. Do not alphabetize; number references in the order in which they are first mentioned in the text. The surnames of the authors followed by initials should be given. There should be no punctuation other than a comma to separate the authors. Cite all authors, 'et al' is not sufficient. Abbreviate journal names according to the Index Medicus system. (Also see International Committee of Medical Journal Editors: Uniform requirements for manuscripts submitted to biomedical journals. Br Med J 1988;296:401-405.)

*Examples*

*(a) Papers published in periodicals:* Kauffman HF, van der Heide S, Beaumont F, Blok H, de Vries K: Class-specific antibody determination against *Aspergillus fumigatus* by means of the enzyme-linked immunosorbent assay. III. Comparative study: IgG, IgA, IgM ELISA titers, precipitating antibodies and IgE binding after fractionation of the antigen. Int Arch Allergy Appl Immunol 1986;80: 300-306.

*(b) Monographs:* Matthews DE, Farewell VT: Using and Understanding Medical Statistics. Basel, Karger, 1985.

*(c) Edited books:* Hardy WD Jr, Essex M: FeLV-induced feline acquired immune deficiency syndrome: A model for human AIDS; in Klein E (ed): Acquired Immunodeficiency Syndrome. Prog Allergy. Basel, Karger, 1986, vol 37, pp 353-376.

*Further details:* Authors may consult our leaflet 'Rules for the Preparation of Manuscripts', available on request from the Publisher, S. Karger AG, P.O. Box, CH-4009 Basel (Switzerland).

**Page charges:** There is no page charge for papers of 4 or fewer printed pages (including tables, illustrations and references). Each additional complete or partial page is charged to the author at SFr. 225.– / US$150.00. The allotted size of a paper is equal to approx. 15 manuscript pages (including tables, illustrations and references).

**Galley proofs:** Unless indicated otherwise, galley proofs are sent to the first-named author and should be returned with the least possible delay. Alterations made in galley proofs, other than the correction of printer's errors, are charged to the author. No page proofs are supplied.

**Reprints:** Order forms and a price list are sent with the galley proofs. Orders submitted after the issue is printed are subject to considerably higher prices. Allow five weeks from date of publication for delivery of reprints.

## General Information


# European Urology

**Publication data:** 'European Urology' is published 8 times annually. Volumes 21–22 with 4 issues each appear in 1992.

**Subscription rates:** Subscriptions run for a full calendar year. Prices are given per volume, surface postage included.

| | |
|---|---|
| *Personal subscription:* | SFr. 289.10, US$ 193.20. |
| (Must be in the name of, billed to, and paid by an individual. Order must be marked 'personal subscription'.) | |
| *Institutional subscription:* | |
| (Regular rate.) | SFr. 413.–, US$ 276.00. |
| *Members* of the European Association of Urology: | SFr. 206.50, US$ 138.00. |
| *Airmail postage:* | SFr. 25.–, US$ 20.00. |
| (Extra per volume.) | |
| *Microform subscription:* | SFr. 206.50, US$ 138.00. |
| (Available exclusively to subscribers of the paper edition.) | |

**Single issues and back volumes:** Information on availability and prices can be obtained through the Publisher.

**Advertising:** Correspondence and rate requests should be addressed to the Publisher.

**Subscription orders:** Orders can be placed at agencies, bookstores, directly with the Publisher S. Karger AG, P.O. Box, CH – 4009 Basel (Switzerland) or with any of the following distributors:

*Deutschland:*
S. Karger GmbH, Lörracher Strasse 16A
Postfach, D-W-7800 Freiburg

*France:* Librairie Luginbühl
36, bd de Latour-Maubourg, F-75007 Paris

*Great Britain, Ireland:*
S. Karger Publishers, 11 Ravenscroft Road
Beckenham, Kent BR3 4TP

*USA:* S. Karger Publishers, Inc.
26 West Avon Road, P.O. Box 529
Farmington, CT 06085

*India, Bangladesh, Sri Lanka:*
S. Karger India Subscription Agency
B – 5/132 Safdarjung Enclave
New Delhi-110029

*Japan:* Katakura Libri, Inc.
36-9 Hongo 3-chome, Bunkyo-ku, Tokyo 113

**Change of address:** Both old and new address should be stated and sent to the subscription source.

**Bibliographic indices:** This journal is regularly listed in bibliographic services, including *Current Contents®*.

**Book Reviews:** Books are accepted for review by special agreement.





KARGER

# Markers in Urology

Proceedings of the
2nd Mediterranean Congress
of Urology,
July 3–6, 1991, Rome, Italy

Guest Editor
*Franco Di Silverio,* Rome

66 figures and 56 tables, 1992

KARGER

**European Urology**
Vol. 21, Supplement 1, 1992

S. Karger
Medical and Scientific Publishers
Basel · Freiburg · Paris · London
New York · New Delhi · Bangkok
Singapore · Tokyo · Sydney

Drug Dosage
The authors and the publisher have exerted every effort to ensure that drug selection and dosage set forth in this text are in accord with current recommendations and practice at the time of publication. However, in view of ongoing research, changes in government regulations, and the constant flow of information relating to drug therapy and drug reactions, the reader is urged to check the package insert for each drug for any change in indications and dosage and for added warnings and precautions. This is particularly important when the recommended agent is a new and/or infrequently employed drug.


P.O. Box, CH–4009 Basel (Switzerland)
Printed in Switzerland on acid-free paper by
Thür AG Offsetdruck, Pratteln
ISBN 3-8055-5612-8

# Table of Contents

Eur Urol 1992;21(suppl 1):1–4

*N. Javadpour*
*R. Guirguis*

University of Maryland and Harbor Hospital Center Baltimore, Md., USA

# Tumor Collagenase-Stimulating Factor and Tumor Autocrine Motility Factor as Tumor Markers in Bladder Cancer – An Update

**Key Words**
Cancer
Bladder
Marker
Enzyme
Urine

**Abstract**
We have studied the role of combined measurements of tumor collagenase-stimulating factor (TCSF) and tumor autocrine motility factor (TAMF) in 83 first morning voids and 24-hour specimens in patients with bladder and renal cancer and control subjects. TCSF and TAMF were measured by immunoabsorption assay and motility test utilizing modified Boyden chamber. The mean concentrations of urinary TCSF and TAMF from cancer patients (n = 32) were 4- to 5-fold higher than those from benign conditions (n = 70). We compared TCSF and TAMF utilizing motility test in first morning voids (n = 18) and 24-hour urinary samples (n = 19). TCSF and TAMF were almost identical in terms of eluted proteins from morning voids and 24-hour urine samples. Invasive bladder cancer (n = 12) showed a significantly higher correlation (r = 0.9 and p = 0.0001) between motility response and urinary concentration of TCSF and TAMF. We have also localized these two glycoproteins in cell membranes and cytoplasms of cancer cell.

Bladder cancer is a group of heterogenous tumors with various natural history and prognostic factors with no reliable tumor marker. The current available biologic markers including ABH, chromosomal analysis, T-antigen, oncofetoproteins, oncogenes and flow cytometry are not frequent and/or specific and sensitive tumor markers for this cancer (table 1) [1, 2].

Tumor-stimulating collagenase factor (TSCF) is a glycoprotein which stimulates fibroblast collagenase production. It is found in urine of bladder cancer patients [3]. Tumor autocrine motility factor (TAMF) is also a cytokine of 54kDa. It is secreted by cancer cells but not secreted by normal and/or inflammatory cells of the urothelium [4, 5].

We have detected and characterized these markers in the urine and cancer cells of patients with bladder cancer. The objective of this communication is to update the technique and results of our 24-hour urine samples from

N. Javadpour, MD
University of Maryland
22 South Greene Street
Baltimore, MD 21201 (USA)


0302–2838/92/0215–0001
$2.75/0

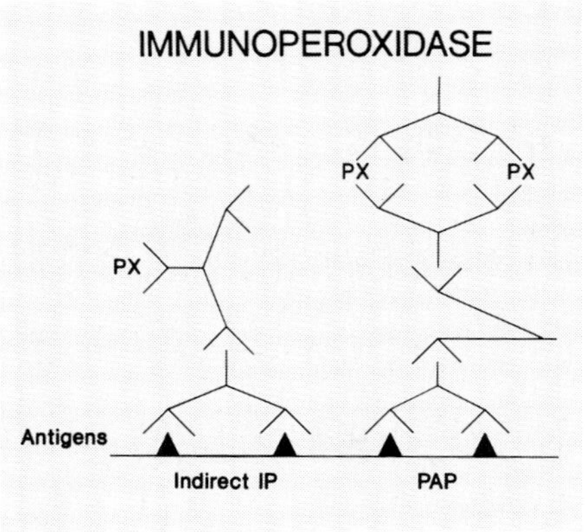


**Fig. 1.** Immunoperoxidase technique.

**Table 1.** Current biologic markers in bladder cancer

| | |
|---|---|
| 1 | ABH isoantigens (RCA, IP) |
| 2 | Chromosomal analysis |
| 3 | T-antigen |
| 4 | DNA, RNA changes in FC |
| 5 | Oncofetal proteins |
| 6 | Oncogene products |

**Table 2.** Processing of 24-hour urine

24-hour urine pH 7.8
↓
Centrifuge 100 ml
↓
Supernatant
↓
Anion exchange beads
↓
Centrifuge the beads
↓
Discard supernatant
↓
Wash twice in PBS
↓
Add 1 ml of eluting buffer

**Table 3.** Motility test

| | |
|---|---|
| 1 | Add sample to lower wells of migration chamber |
| 2 | Utilizing type IV collagen-coated membrane |
| 3 | Add cells to upper wells |
| 4 | Incubate for 4 h |
| 5 | Fix and stain |
| 6 | Read the color on densitometer |

patients with bladder cancer and localization of these markers in transitional and squamous cell carcinoma of the bladder.

## Materials and Methods

*Urine Collection*

Twenty-four (24) hour and early morning urine specimens were collected from bladder cancer patients, normal volunteers, patients with various inflammatory and/or other genitourinary cancers.

*Preparation of Urine for Motility Assay*

For the motility assay, the eluted sample solution was processed further as follows: 0.9 ml of the eluted protein solution from the shuttle was concentrated to 100 ml using a microconcentrator with molecular weight cut-off of 30 kDa by centrifugation at 3,750 rpm for 6 min (table 2). A modified migration chamber coated with type IV collagen membrane is utilized to detect motility factor as previously reported (table 3). The conventional enzyme-linked immunoabsorption assay ELISA method was utilized to detect TCSF and TAMF in urine of patients with bladder cancer.

*Immunohistochemical Techniques*

The technique of immunohistochemical detection of TAMF and TCSF have previously been discussed (fig. 1). Monoclonal antibodies are raised against the TCSF and TAMF and utilized for immunohistological staining of both transitional and squamous cell carcinoma.

## Results

We compared the amounts of TCSF, TAMF, and motility response in first morning voids (18 patients) and 24-hour urine samples (19 patients). The levels of TCSF and TAMF concentrations were almost identical in the eluted samples from morning voids and 24-hour urines. This suggests that first morning voids can be used as sample source to detect the presence or absence of these markers. The motility response, however, was inconsistent.

*Invasive and Noninvasive Bladder Cancer*

To see if there is any correlation between invasiveness of the tumor and the level of TCSF, TAMF, and the motility response in the eluted samples, we used multiple regression analysis which was performed on test-positive patients. Genitourinary cancer cases with invasive tumors (12 patients) showed a significantly high correlaton ($r = 0.9$, $p = 0.001$) between motility response (dependent variable) versus TCSF and TAMF concentrations (independent variables). While, in the case of noninvasive tumors, there were no correlations between the motility

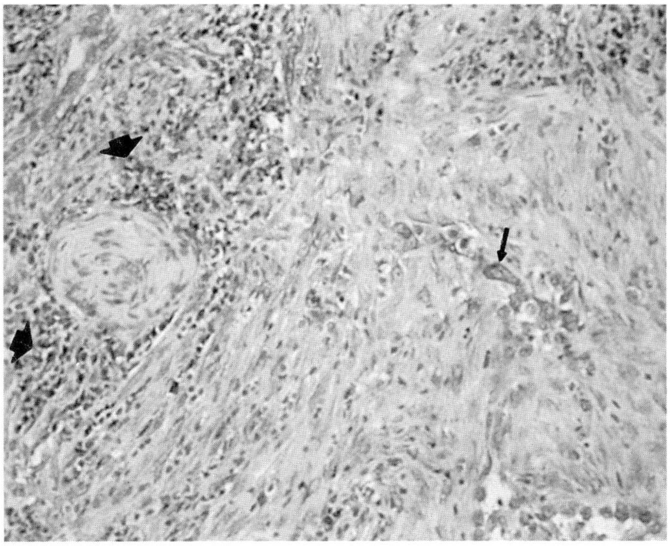

**Fig. 2.** Immunohistochemical staining of cancer cells of the bladder utilizing antibody to the TAMF. Note the infiltrating cancer cell staining (arrow) but the inflammatory cells are not staining (arrowheads).

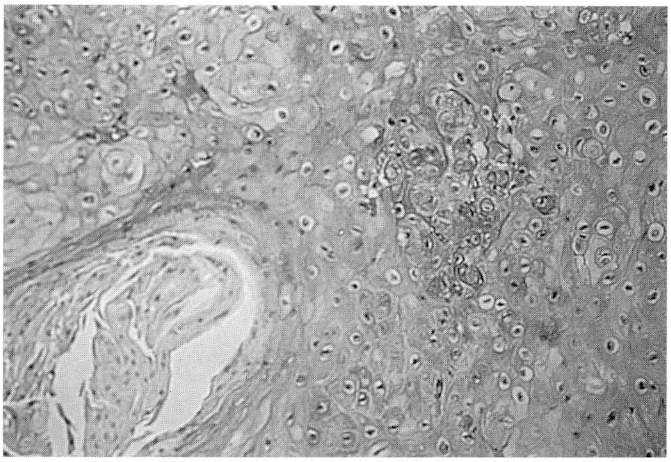

**Fig. 3.** Squamous cell carcinoma immunostained utilizing monoclonal antibody to TCSF.

values and the amount of TCSF and TAMF present in the samples.

In the preoperative bladder cancer patients, the mean concentration values of TCSF (329.2 ± 94.1) and TAMF (290 ± 81.2) were significantly higher than the postoperative patients (182.9 ± 81.2) and (166.7 ± 55.4) consecutive.

## Discussion

Bladder cancer is a group of heterogenous tumors with variable natural histories and prognostic outcomes. This cancer has no known reliable tumor marker at the present time. In search of identifying such a marker, we have detected the urinary and cellular TCSF and TAMF in patients with bladder cancer and other malignancies [5]. TCSF is membrane-bound glycoprotein of tumor cell which stimulates fibroblast collagen production. TAMF is a 70-kD glycoprotein secreted by malignant cell and is responsible for cell locomotion. We have studied the role of combined measurements of TCSF and TAMF in 83 first morning voids and 24-hour specimens in patients with bladder and renal cancer and control subjects. All urine samples were processed at 4 °C and obtaining their eluted proteins from the samples. TCSF and TAMF were measured by immunoabsorption assay and motility test utilizing modified Boyden chamber. The mean concentrations of urinary TCSF and TAMF from cancer patients (n = 32) were 4- to 5-fold higher than those from benign conditions (n = 70). We compared TCSF and TAMF utilizing motility test in first morning voids (n = 18) and 24-hour urinary samples (n = 19). TCSF and TAMF were almost identical in terms of eluted proteins from morning voids and 24-hour urine samples. Invasive bladder cancer (n = 12) showed a significantly higher correlation (r = 0.9) and p = 0.0001) between motility response and urinary concentration of TCSF and TAMF. For noninvasive tumors, there was no correlation between the motility values and the amount of eluted TCSF and TAMF. We have also localized these two glycoproteins in cell membranes and cytoplasms of cancer cell. The TCSF is localized in membrane of the transitional cell carcinoma, as well as squamous cell carcinoma of the bladder, utilizing monoclonal antibodies to these markers.

Currently we are studying the prospective role of these markers in detecting recurrent bladder cancer, monitoring the therapy and forecasting the progress of patients with bladder cancer.

*In conclusion:* TCSF and TAMF are glycoproteins that are synthesized by cancer cells of patients with bladder cancer. These tumor markers are excreted in urine by the cancer cells of the bladder tumor. TCSF and TAMF are detected in urine of bladder cancer patients utilizing

ELISA and a modified migration chamber coated with type IV collagenase membrane (fig. 2, 3). These markers are significantly elevated in urine of patients with bladder cancer having a good correlation (r = 0.8). TCSF and TAMF are localized in tumor cells of patients with bladder cancer utilizing specific and sensitive antibodies raised against these glycoproteins. These markers are being studied prospectively for monitoring the therapy, detecting the recurrence and forecasting the prognosis of patients with bladder cancer.

## References


1 Javadpour N: Multiple cell markers in bladder cancer. Principles and clinical applications. Urol Clin North Am 1984;11:609–616.
2 Davidsohn I: Early immunologic diagnosis and prognosis of carcinoma. Am J Clin Pathol 1972;57:715.
3 Biswas C, Bloch KJ, Gross J: Collagenolytic activity of rabbit V2 carcinoma implanted in the nude mouse. JNCI 1982;69:1329–1336.
4 Liotta LA, Mandler R, Murano G, Katz DA, Gordon RK, Chiang PK, Schiffmann E: Tumor cell autocrine motility factor. Proc Natl Acad Sci USA 1986;83:3302–3306.
5 Guirguis R, Margulies I, Taraboletti G, et al: Cytokine-induced pseudopodial protrusion is coupled to tumor cell migration. Nature 1987;329:261–263.

Eur Urol 1992;21(suppl 1):5–9

M.C. Sanchez-Fernandez de Sevilla[a]
L. Morell-Quadreny[a]
M. Gil-Salom[b]
M. Perez-Bacete[a]
A. Llombart-Bosch[a]

[a] Department of Pathology (Prof. *A. Llombart-Bosch*) and
[b] Service of Urology (Department of Surgery), University Medical School, Valencia, Spain

# Morphometric and Immunohistochemical Characterization of Bladder Carcinoma in situ and Its Preneoplastic Lesions

**Key Words**
Bladder cancer
Carcinoma in situ
Urothelial dysplasia
Morphometry
Immunochemistry
Lectins
Epithelial differentiation antigens
Blood group isoantigens

**Abstract**
We performed a morphometric and immunohistochemical study of 26 bladder carcinoma in situ (Cis) specimens, compared with normal urothelium and urothelial preneoplastic lesions. The following morphometric parameters were evaluated: nuclear area, nuclear perimeter and maximum nuclear diameter. For the immunohistochemical study we used five lectins, antibodies against four epithelial differentiation antigens, and antibodies against blood group isoantigens.

A progressive increase in nuclear size from normal urothelium to dysplastic urothelium and Cis was detected. Nuclear size values in Cis and in high-grade, high-stage bladder carcinomas were similar. The most relevant immunohistochemical results were obtained with CEA, CK, UEA-1 and ABH isoantigens, which show significant immunoreactivity changes in preneoplastic urothelium and Cis when compared with normal urothelium.

We conclude that bladder Cis behaves morphometrically and immunohistochemically as an invasive bladder carcinoma, and we emphasize the usefulness of these techniques for detecting flat dysplastic and neoplastic lesions in random bladder biopsies.

## Introduction

It is well known that, at presentation, 70–75% of patients with bladder cancer have superficial tumors, that 70% of them will recur, and that 10–15% of recurrences are invasive carcinomas. The remaining 25–30% of patients with bladder cancer have tumors that are already high-grade, high-stage invasive carcinomas at presentation.

In this study we evaluate the hypothesis that bladder carcinoma in situ (Cis) is the source of these 25–30% rapidly invasive carcinomas. This concept was formerly proposed by the authors who described Cis [1–4], who consider Cis as an 'anaplasia of the surface epithelium without the formation of papillary structures and without infiltration', so reflecting its malignant and invasive potential.

In order to support this concept we have performed a morphometric and immunohistochemical study of 26 bladder Cis specimens, primitive or associated with exophytic tumor, compared with normal urothelium and other preneoplastic lesions.

Carmen Sanchez-Fernandez de Sevilla, MD
Department of Pathology, Faculty of Medicine
Av. Blasco Ibanez, 17
E-46010 Valencia (Spain)


0302–2838/92/0215–0005
$2.75/0

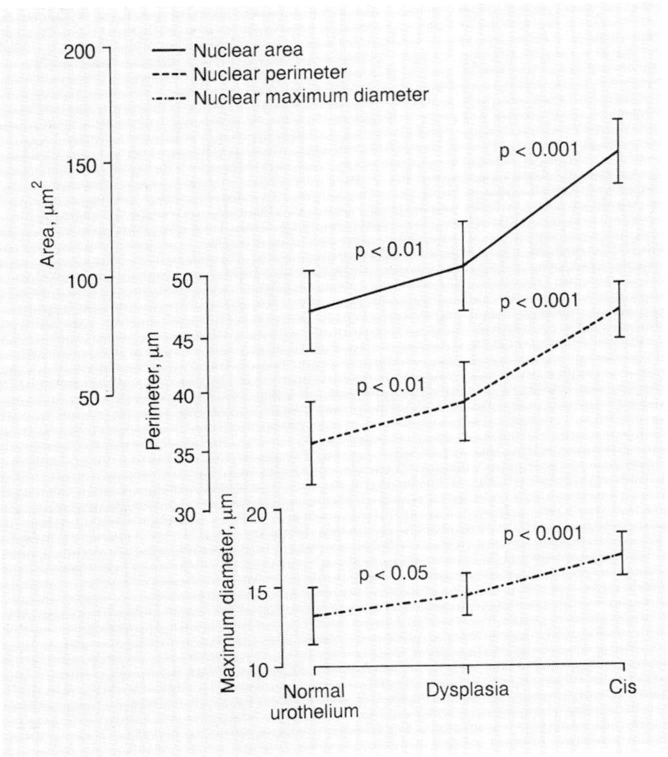


**Fig. 1.** Morphometric results in normal urothelium, dysplastic urothelium and Cis.

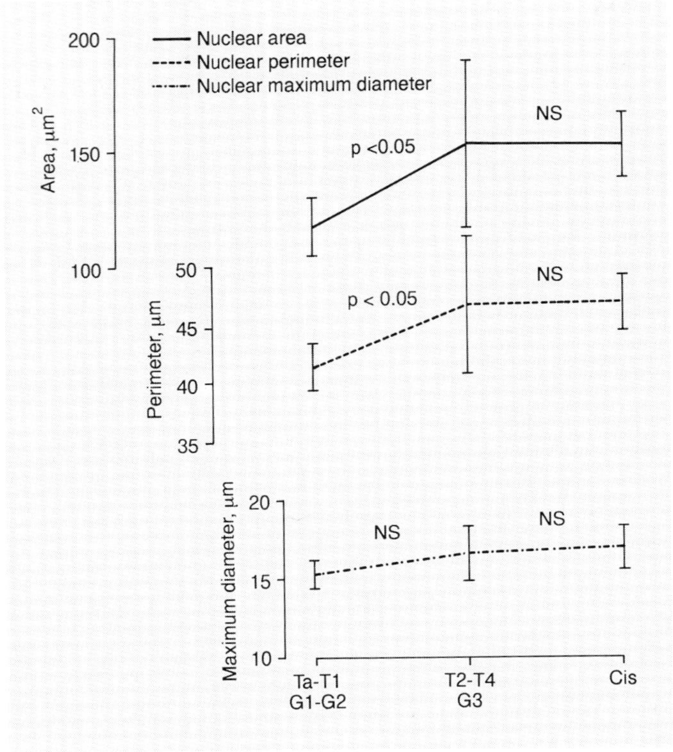


**Fig. 2.** Morphometric results in bladder carcinomas vs. Cis. Nuclear area Ta-T1, G1-G2 tumors vs. Cis: $p < 0.001$. Nuclear perimeter Ta-T1, G1-G2 tumors vs. Cis: $p < 0.001$. Maximum nuclear diameter Ta-T1, G1-G2 tumors vs. Cis: $p < 0.05$. NS: not significant.

## Material and Methods

One hundred and four bladder tumors, obtained from 78 patients, were studied (93 males, 11 females, mean age 67 years, range 23–78). Forty cases were superficial, low-grade tumors (Ta-T1, G1-G2) obtained by TUR. Thirty-two cases were invasive high grade tumors (T2-T4, G3) obtained by radical cystectomy. In 26 of them, the previous TUR specimen was also studied. The remaining 6 cases were autopsy specimens from patients who died with metastatic bladder cancer without cystectomy.

Histologically normal urothelium (30 specimens), urothelial dysplasia (13 specimens) and Cis (26 specimens) were obtained from flat, macroscopically normal-looking mucosa from cystectomy specimens.

Morphometric study was performed measuring 300 nuclei from representative tumor areas, previously photographed in black and white at 1,000×. Nuclear area, nuclear perimeter and maximum nuclear diameter were measured with an image analysis system (MOP-Videoplan 2000, Zeiss-Kontron).

Immunohistochemical study was performed with five lectins: concanavalin A (Con-A, 10 μg/ml; Sigma), wheat germ agglutinin (WGA, 25 μg/ml; Sigma), soybean agglutinin (SBA; 12.5 μg/ml; Sigma), *Ulex europaeus* gorse type 1 (UEA-1, 2 μg/ml; Sigma) and peanut agglutinin (PNA, 5 μg/ml; Sigma), the latter with and without pretreatment with neuraminidase (0.01 U/ml; Sigma). An indirect, immunoperoxidase two-step method was used, as proposed by Nakane [5].

The pattern of immunoreactivity of four epithelial differentiation antigens was studied with two polyclonal antibodies – panepithelial Keratin (K; Dako) and carcinoembryonic antigen (CEA; Dako) – using the PAP method [6] and two monoclonal antibodies – simple epithelium cytokeratin (CK; Dako) and epithelial membrane antigen (EMA; Dako) – using the ABC method [7]. The following dilutions of antibodies were used: anti-CEA: 1/750; anti-K: 1/300; anti-CK: 1/100, and anti-EMA: 1/200. Expression of ABH blood group isoantigens was also studied with monoclonal antibodies (A: 1/50; B: 1/50; H: 1/50), employing the ABC method [7].

Immunohistochemical results were expressed as intensity of immunostaining, graded as negative (–), poorly positive (+), moderately positive (++) or strongly positive (+++).

For statistical evaluation of morphometric results, t test was used.

**Table 1.** Lectins

| | UEA-1 | PNA | PNA+N | CON-A | SBA | WGA |
|---|---|---|---|---|---|---|
| Normal urothelium | | | | | | |
| Superficial layer | +++ | – | + | + | – | ++ |
| Intermediate layer | – | – | + | + | – | ++ |
| Basal layer | – | – | + | + | – | ++ |
| Dysplastic urothelium | ++ | – | +/– | + | – | ++ |
| Carcinoma in situ | +++ | +/– | – | + | – | ++ |
| Superficial tumors | +++ | +/– | ++ | ++ | – | ++ |
| Invasive tumors | +++ | + | – | ++ | +/– | ++ |

**Table 2.** Epithelial differentiation antigens and blood group isoantigens

| | CEA | K | CK | EMA | A | B | H |
|---|---|---|---|---|---|---|---|
| Normal urothelium | | | | | | | |
| Superficial layer | +/– | +/– | – | ++ | +++ | +++ | +++ |
| Intermediate layer | +/– | +/– | – | + | +++ | +++ | +++ |
| Basal layer | +/– | +/– | ++ | – | +++ | +++ | +++ |
| Dysplastic urothelium | + | +/– | + | + | ++ | ++ | ++ |
| Carcinoma in situ | ++ | +/– | +/– | +/– | – | – | – |
| Superficial tumors | ++ | ++ | + | +/– | ++ | ++ | +++ |
| Invasive tumors | +++ | ++ | + | + | +/– | +/– | +/– |

## Results

When comparing nuclear size (area, perimeter and diameter) in normal urothelium, dysplastic urothelium and Cis, a progressive increase in these parameters was observed (fig. 1).

Nuceli of superficial tumors were significantly smaller than nuclei of Cis. No significant differences, however, were found in nuclear size of invasive tumors and Cis (fig. 2).

The most significant immunohistochemical results with lectins were obtained with UEA-1 and PNA. In normal urothelium, *Ulex* stains selectively the superficial cells, but in Cis and in invasive tumors, UEA-1 is positive in the entire urothelial thickness. In superficial tumors, UEA-1 positivity and distribution is irregular (table 1).

Normal urothelium does not stain with PNA, whereas in dysplastic urothelium and in Cis a progressive increase in staining with this lectin is observed. When sections were pretreated with neuraminidase (PNA+N), reactivity to PNA does invert. Staining, with this lectin in superficial tumors behaves as in normal urothelium, and in invasive tumors does so as in Cis (table 1).

Other lectins used in this study did not reveal significant changes, being basically positive Con-A and WGA and negative SBA.

The most relevant results with epithelial differentiation antigens were obtained with CEA and CK. CEA is poorly positive in normal urothelium and becomes progressively more positive in dysplasia and Cis. CK presents a specific staining pattern in the basal layer of normal urothelium, this pattern being lost in Cis, where it is poorly positive in the whole epithelial thickness (table 2).

Blood group isoantigens are positive in normal urothelium, but become progressively more negative in dysplasia and in Cis. Blood group isoantigens behave in superficial tumors as in normal urothelium, being positive in the totality of cells, while invasive tumors lose this positivity, like Cis (table 2).

## Discussion

Cis is considered as a superficial bladder cancer, with a variable macroscopic appearance [1–3], and often multifocal [4]. The time taken for progression from in situ to invasive carcinoma has been reported to be variable (10–70 months) [4]. Patients with superficial bladder cancer who present Cis or other mucosal abnormalities in random biopsies of macroscopically normal-looking bladder mucosa have been reported to be more prone to develop tumor recurrences and progression to invasive cancer [8–10]. Dalla et al. [11] termed urinary intraepithelial neoplasia (UIA) the spectrum of bladder intraepithelial changes between normal urothelium and frank carcinoma, which would represent different steps of the same process leading to bladder cancer.

In the present study we have not established different grades in this variety of preneoplastic lesions, which were grouped together under the term 'dysplasia', since a more accurate classification has no, in practice, therapeutic implications. Dysplasia has been, however, distinguished from frank Cis, since the latter demands a more active therapeutic attitude.

Significant changes in nuclear size in preneoplastic bladder lesions have been reported, which correlate with variations in DNA content [12–14]. Our study confirms these changes and highlights the morphometric analogy between Cis and high-grade, high-stage carcinomas, and the morphometric differences between Cis and superficial carcinomas.

A progressive increase in staining for CEA in dysplasia and Cis was one of the most significant findings in our study. Wahren [15] noted that normal urothelial cells did not express CEA, but in the vicinity of papillary tumors, CEA-positive cell populations were identified. These did not differ morphologically from normal, CEA-negative, urothelium. Shevchuk et al. [16] reported that CEA is present in normal urothelium, without significant changes in Cis.

In our study CEA shows a specific staining pattern for superficial cells in superficial tumors, while in invasive tumors the totality of cells express this antigen. A progressive increase in the number of CEA-positive tumors with higher grade and stage has also been reported [17–19].

CK shows in our study a specific staining pattern for the basal layer of normal urothelium. CK positivity extends in dysplasia and Cis to the remaining epithelial layers. In superficial tumors, CK expression is similar to normal urothelium. Most invasive tumors are CK-negative, but some of them, mainly those with high nucleus/cytoplasm ration, are CK-positive. Ramaekers et al. [20] found with CK-18 a selective staining pattern for superficial cells in normal urothelium and well-differentiated tumors, while in some invasive tumors all the cells are CK-positive.

EMA and panepithelial keratin were basically positive both in normal and in neoplastic urothelium, in agreement with the findings of other authors [20–23].

The only lectin that shows a specific staining pattern in normal urothelium is UEA-1, being positive in the luminal surface of superficial cells. This positivity extends to other cell layers in dysplastic urothelium, and to the whole epithelial thickness in Cis. In some cases, an irregular immunostaining with UEA-1 was observed in 'apparently normal' urothelium areas, a finding also reported by Coon and Weinstein [24] and whose interpretation is uncertain. Both in superficial and in invasive transitional carcinomas, immunostaining with UEA-1 is also irregular in distribution.

Results with blood group isoantigens were similar in Cis and in invasive tumors. Expression of these antigens by tumors, however, is not an all-or-nothing feature [25]. In some specimens there were areas both positive and negative.

We conclude that Cis behaves morphometrically and immunohistochemically as an invasive bladder carcinoma, supporting the concept that it is the principal source of invasive cancer. Moreover, morphometric and immunohistochemical techniques allow a more objective characterization of urothelial dysplasia and carcinoma in situ than routine histological evaluation.

## References


1 De Voogt HJ, Rathert R, Beyer-Boon ME: In situ carcinoma; in De Voogt HJ, Rathert R, Beyer-Boon ME (eds): Urinary Cytology. Berlin, Springer, 1977, pp 127–133.

2 Melicow MM, Hollowell JW: Intraurothelial cancer: Carcinoma in situ. Bowen's disease of the urinary system: Discussion of thirty cases. J Urol 1952;68:763–772.

3 Umiker W, Lapides J, Sourenne R: Exfoliative cytology of papillomas and intraepithelial carcinomas of the urinary bladder. Acta Cytol 1962;6:255–260.

4 Melamed MD, Voutsa NC, Grabstald M: Natural history and clinical behavior of in situ carcinoma of the human urinary bladder. Cancer 1964;17:1533–1545.

5 Nakane PK: Simultaneous localization of multiple tissue antigens using the peroxidase-labeled antibody method. A study on the pituitary gland of the rat. J Histochem Cytochem 1968;16:557–560.

6 Sternberger LA, Hardy PH, Cuculis JJ, Meyer HG: The unlabeled antibody enzyme method of immunohistochemistry. Preparation and properties of soluble antigen antibody complex (horseradish-peroxidase antihorseradish-peroxidase) and its use in identification of spirochetes. J Histochem Cytochem 1970;16:315–333.

7 Hsu SM, Raine L, Fanger H: Use of avidin-biotin-peroxidase complex (ABC) in immunoperoxidase techniques: A comparison between ABC and unlabeled antibody (PAP) procedures. J Histochem Cytochem 1981;29:577–580.

8 Eisenberg RL, Roth RB, Schweinsberg MH: Bladder tumors and associated proliferative mucosal lesions. J Urol 1960;84:540–550.

9 Althausen A, Prout GR, Daly JJ: Non-invasive papillary carcinoma of bladder associated with carcinoma in situ. J Urol 1976;116:576–579.

10 Koss LG: Tumors of the urinary bladder. Washington, Armed Forces Institute of Pathology, 1975.

11 Dalla PP, Parenti A, De Caro E, Piazza M: Urinary intraepithelial neoplasia. Pathol Res Pract 1984;178:121–127.

12 Helander K, Hofer P, Holmberg G: Karyometric investigations on urinary bladder carcinoma, correlated to histopathological grading. Virchows Arch [A] 1984;403:117–125.

13 Gustafson H, Tribukait B, Brehmer-Endersson E: Detection of different DNA stem cell lines in a case of human bladder carcinoma. Acta Pathol Microbiol Scand [A] 1981;89:133–135.

14 Klein FA, Herr HW, Sogani PC, Whitmore WF, Melamed MR: Flow cytometry of normal and non-neoplastic diseases of the bladder: an estimate of the false-positive rate. J Urol 1982; 127:946–948.

15 Wahren B: Cellular content of carcinoembryonic antigen in urothelial carcinoma. Cancer 1978;42:1533–1539.

16 Shevchuk MM, Fenoglio CM, Richart RM: Carcinoembryonic antigen localization in benign and malignant transitional epithelium. Cancer 1981;47:899–905.

17 Wiley EL, Mendelsohn G, Droller MJ, Eggleston JC: Immunoperoxidase detection of carcinoembryonic antigen and blood group substances in papillary transitional cell carcinoma of the bladder. J Urol 1982;128:276–280.

18 Jautzke G, Altenaher E: Immunohistochemical demonstration of carcinoembryonic antigen and its correlation with grading and staging on tissue sections of urinary bladder carcinomas. Cancer 1982;50:2052–2056.

19 López-Beltrán A, Garcia-Calvo J, Morales C, Fanego J, Molina I, Toro-Rojas H: Determinación inmunohistoquímica del antígeno carcinoembrionario en carcinomas uroteliales de vejiga. Oncología 1986;9:44–48.

20 Ramaekers F, Huysman A, Muesker D, Schaart G, Herman CH, Vooijs P: Cytokeratin expression during neoplastic progression of human transitional cell carcinomas as detected by a monoclonal and polyclonal antibody. Lab Invest 1985;52:31–38.

21 Pinkus GS, Kurtin PJ: Epithelial membrane antigen – A diagnostic discriminant in surgical pathology: Immunohistochemical profile in epithelial, mesenchymal and hematopoietic neoplasms using paraffin sections and monoclonal antibodies. Hum Pathol 1985;16:929–940.

22 Heyderman E, Brown BH, Richardson TC: Epithelial markers in prostatic, bladder, and colorectal cancer: an immunoperoxidase study of epithelial membrane antigen, carcinoembryonic antigen, and prostatic acid phosphatase. J Clin Pathol 1984;37:1363–1369.

23 Said JW: Immunohistochemical localization of keratin proteins in tumor diagnosis. Hum Pathol 1983;14:1017–1019.

24 Coon JS, Weinstein RS: Detection of ABH tissue isoantigens by immunoperoxidase methods in normal and neoplastic urothelium. Comparison with the erythrocyte adherence method. Am J Clin Pathol 1981;76:163–171.

25 Weinstein RS, Coon J, Alroy J, Davidsohn I: Tissue-associated blood group antigens in human tumors; in De Lellis RA (ed): Diagnostic Immunochemistry. New York, Masson, 1981, pp 239–261.

Eur Urol 1992;21(suppl 1):10–12

*A. Schmidt*
*P. Bub*
*U. Rüther*
*F. Eisenberger*

Department of Urology, Katharinenhospital, Stuttgart, FRG

# Tissue Polypeptide Antigen for Monitoring of Advanced Bladder Cancer after MVEC Chemotherapy

**Key Words**
Tissue polypeptide antigen
Advanced bladder cancer
MVEC chemotherapy

**Abstract**
58 patients with advanced bladder cancer were treated with MVEC chemotherapy (methotrexate, vinblastine, epirubicin and cisplatinum). 22 patients suffered from locally advanced disease (pT3–4 M0 N0), in 20 patients regional lymph node metastases were found (pT3–4 N1–3 M0). In 16 patients distant metastases were noted (pT1–4 N0–1 M1). In 89% transitional cell and in 11% squamous cell cancer or anaplastic carcinoma was seen. Complete response was noted in 45%, partial response in 23% and no response in 32%. Tissue polypeptide antigen (TPA) was registered before each course of chemotherapy and 3 months after the last application. The sensitivity for (pT3–4 N0 M0) tumors was 90.9%, for (pT3–4 N1–3 M0) 100% and for tumors with distant metastases 100% also, overall 96,6%. No statistically significant different values between each tumor group were found. In 85,7% a concordant reaction of TPA values and clinical status was notable. In conclusion, TPA has been proven as a valuable and a reliable marker for monitoring therapeutic efficacy of chemotherapy for advanced bladder cancer.

## Introduction

The prognosis of advanced bladder cancer has to be considered poor, since radiotherapy and radical surgery have not fulfilled their expectations yet. In the days of modern polychemotherapy of advanced bladder cancer this pessimistic view has to be changed, as long-term complete responses were reported [1]. Since the chemotherapy is combined with even life-threatening toxicity, a modality to detect insufficient response or tumor recurrency as soon as possible is necessary. Unfortunately no tumor marker system has been established for bladder cancer yet. Based on investigations of Björklund and Björklund [2] in 1957, who described a tumor-associated membrane protein with a molecular weight of 45,000 daltons, tissue polypeptide antigen (TPA) has been used as a tumor marker for bladder cancer since 1975 [3]. We would like to present our experience with this tumor marker system for monitoring of the chemotherapy of advanced bladder cancer.

Dr. A. Schmidt
Urologische Klinik, Katharinenhospital
Postfach 102644
D-W-7000 Stuttgart 10 (FRG)


0302–2838/92/0215–0010
$2.75/0

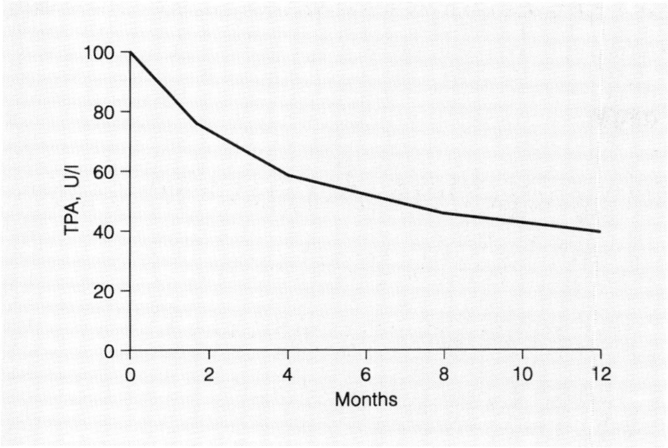


**Fig. 1.** Case 1 (see text for details).

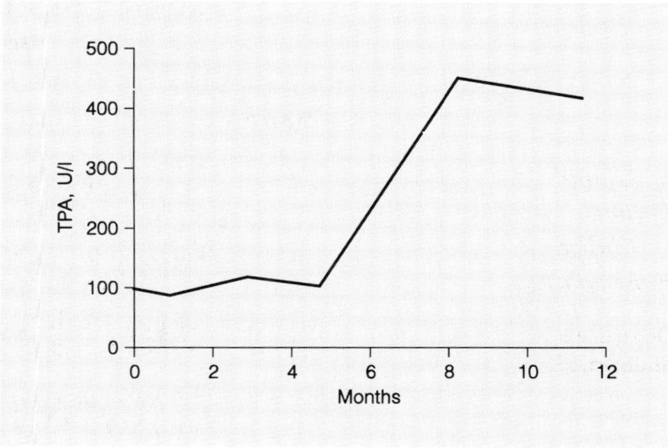


**Fig. 2.** Case 2 (see text for details).

## Material and Methods

58 patients, 46 men and 12 women, with a mean age of 65.3 years, suffering from advanced bladder cancer, received on average 3.9 courses of polychemotherapy of the MVEC regimen consisting of 30 mg/m$^2$ methotrexate, 3 mg/m$^2$ vinblastine, 70 mg/m$^2$ cisplatinum and 30 mg/m$^2$ 4-epirubicin. Minimal follow-up was 12 months with a mean follow-up of 22 months. 22 patients (37,1%) had organ-confined disease (pT3–4 N0 M0). 20 patients (33.4%) suffered from regional disease (pT3–4 N1–3 M0) and 16 patients (27.7%) had distant metastases (pT1–4 N0–1 M1). Distant metastases were found in the lung in 4 cases and distant lymph nodes in 3 patients, bone, liver and skin metastases were seen in 3 cases each. 52 patients (89.6%) had pure transitional cell carcinoma. In 5 patients (8.6%) squamous cell carcinoma was seen and in 1 patient anaplastic carcinoma was found. All 22 patients with organ-confined disease had only TUR B before the chemotherapy. 14 patients with regional disease had TUR and 6 were treated after cystectomy in an adjuvant fashion. 9 patients with distant metastases had TUR B only, while in 8 patients cystectomy was performed before.

TPA values were measured before the chemotherapy, after each course and in 3-monthly intervals. Analysis was performed with the Prolifigen TPA IRMA test kit (Sangtec Medical, Bromma, Sweden). The lower detection threshold was evaluated with 5 U/l, the 95th percentile of 353 healthy blood donors was registered at 50 U/l.

## Results

Of 22 patients with organ-confined disease (T1–4 N0 M0) TPA was elevated in 20 cases (sensitivity 90.9%) with mean values of 93.9 ± 36.7 U/l. In 20 patients with lymph node metastases (T1–4 N1 M0) TPA was elevated in all cases (sensitivity 100%) with mean values of 121.7 ± 43.7 U/l. In 16 patients with distant metastases (T1–4 N0–1 M1) TPA was elevated in all cases (sensitivity 100%) with mean values of 156.3 ± 62.5 U/l. Overall sensitivity of TPA was 96.6%.

A gradual trend to higher TPA values was notable with more extended and progressed disease, although no statistically significant difference was found ($p > 0.1$).

The retrospective stratification depending on response to chemotherapy revealed initial TPA values for 26 complete responders of 120 ± 35 U/l, for partial responders of 149 ± 49 U/l (n = 13) and for 19 nonresponders of 183 ± 64 U/l. Although not statistically significant also ($p > 0.1$), high TPA levels before chemotherapy indicated large tumor burden and poor prognosis.

After complete clinical response after MVEC chemotherapy, TPA dropped to normal values (< 50 U/l) in 22 of 26 patients (84%). In case of stable disease or partial response, TPA remained stable in 90.4% (19 of 21 patients). In 10 of 11 cases with tumor progression, TPA increased too (90.9%). Overall concordance to clinical performance status was found in 87.1%.

## Case Reports

*Case 1:* A 53-year-old male patient with invasive bladder cancer (pT3 N0 M0 G2–3) had significant reduction of TPA from 100 to 70 U/l after the first course. During a follow-up of 14 months, normal values were achieved and still indicated complete response (fig. 1).

*Case 2:* A 66-year-old male patient with invasive bladder cancer (pT2 N2 M0 G2–3) received chemotherapy after pelvine staging lymphadenectomy and radical cystectomy in an adjuvant fashion. During 4 courses of MVEC, TPA remained between 99 and 125 U/l. After chemotherapy, TPA increased up to 470 U/l. Bone metastases and local recurrence were diagnosed simultaneously (fig. 2).

## Discussion

Although TPA was described already in 1957, it has not been established as a tumor marker system for bladder cancer. Regarding the current literature indicating a sensitivity of 92% at a specificity of 95% [4], TPA remains the only useful marker for this tumor entity. After MVEC chemotherapy, similar sensitivity was found in our group of patients. Simultaneous immunohistochemical investigations revealed that TPA was detectable in almost all urethelial cancers [5].

During MVEC chemotherapy the correlation between the TPA values and the clinical performance status was of major interest to detect insufficient response at the earliest possible moment. The TPA values of complete responders differed from those of nonresponders at a high statistical level. Therefore, TPA can signalize the reduction of tumor mass after chemotherapy significantly: on the other hand, no response or early tumor recurrence can be detected, and therapeutic alternatives have to be offered.

## Conclusion

TPA has been established as an ideal marker for monitoring of patients with advanced bladder cancer during chemotherapy, because of its high specificity, sensitivity and correlation to clinical status.

## References


1 Sternberg CN, Yagoda A, Scher HI, Watson RC, Tarseef A, Weeiselberg LR, Geller N, Hollander PS, Herr HW, Sogani PC, Morse MJ, Whitmore WF: Preliminary results of M-VAC (methotrexate, vinblastine, doxorubicin and cisplatin) for transitional cell carcinoma of the urothelium. J Urol 1985;133:403–407.

2 Björklund B, Björklund V: Antigenicity of pooled human malignant and normal tissue by cytoimmunological technique: Presence of an insoluble, heat-labile tumor antigen. Int Arch Allergy 1957;10:153–184.

3 Menendez-Botet CJ, Oettgen HF, Pinsky CM, Schwartz MK: A preliminary evaluation of tissue polypeptide antigen in serum or urine (or both) of patients with cancer or benign neoplasms. Clin Chem 1978;24:868–872.

4 Adolphs H-D, Oehr P: Significance of plasma tissue polypeptide antigen determination for diagnosis and follow-up of urothelial bladder cancer. Urol Res 1984;12:125–128.

5 Vogel J, Oehr P: Immunhistochemischer Nachweis von TPA und CEA in menschlichen Geweben und Tumoren; in Lüthgens M, Schlegel G (eds): Tumormarkersystem CEA-TPA. Leonberg, Tumor-Diagnostik Verlag, 1987, pp 47–60.

Eur Urol 1992;21(suppl 1):13–15

*J. Romero*
*L. Alos*
*C. Mallofre*
*M. Sole*
*R. Gutierrez*
*J. Alcover*
*P. Carretero*

Departments of Urology and Pathology, University of Barcelona, Hospital Clinic, Barcelona, Spain

# Bladder Wash Cytology and Flow Cytometry for the Diagnosis of Transitional Cell Carcinoma of the Urinary Bladder

**Key Words**
Bladder wash cytology
Flow cytometry
Bladder cancer

**Abstract**
The role of bladder wash (BW) cytology and flow cytometry in the diagnosis of low-grade transitional cell carcinoma (TCC) of the bladder is yet to be demonstrated. We have studied a series of BW specimens by both conventional cytology and flow cytometry: there were 16 BW from patients with histologically proven TCC and 14 BW from patients with clinical suspicion of tumor or under follow-up for previous TCC in which no evidence of tumor was found by cystoscopy and multiple biopsies. As control group, 21 BW were studied from patients undergoing cystoscopy for causes other than TCC.

In conclusion, the conventional cytologic study of BW specimens was highly sensitive for grade II–III TCC, but missed most grade I TCC; flow cytometric analysis did not improve significantly the detection rate in low-grade TCC.

## Introduction

Traditionally, cystoscopy with the aid of classical urinary cytology have been the basic tools for the follow-up of superficial bladder carcinoma. Urinary cytology has been used since 1940 with the Papanicolau technique, attributing to it a mean number of diagnoses of 70% in bladder cancer, with large variations according to the degree of tumor [1, 2]. Other additional factors such as urinary infections, endocavity treatments or lithiasis lessen cytology reliability even more (and also that of cystoscopy [3]. Furthermore, the subjectivity of the pathologist in assigning the degree of tumor has been widely demonstrated [4–6]. This is very important if we take into account that the degree of tumor is still currently a fundamental factor in prognosis [7]. In this context, the appearance a few years ago fo an automated technique for determining cell DNA, such as flow cytometry, has opened up new perspectives in the diagnosis, prognosis and follow-up of bladder cancer. However, its application in the everyday clinical situation still has to be determined [8].

In numerous studies flow cytometry has shown a diagnostic sensitivity of over 85% [9–13] in TCC and the greater number of recurrences and progressions in aneuploid tumors compared with the better prognosis of euploid ones appears to be indisputable [14, 15]. In this study, our aim is to evaluate by comparison cytology and flow cytometry of bladder wash (BW) in the diagnosis of low-degree transitional cell carcinoma (TCC).

J. Romero
Department of Urology, University of Barcelona
Hospital Clinic, Villarroel, 170
E–08036 Barcelona (Spain)


0302–2838/92/0215–0013
$2.75/0

## Patients and Methods

We performed BW with saline solution (100 $cm^3$) by means of Ellick's evacuator, at the time of performing a cystoscopy. The specimen was split, with half sent for cytology and half for flow cytometry studies. The specimens were refrigerated immediately and processed within 12 h.

BW specimens were obtained from 51 patients divided into 3 groups: (A) 16 patients with superficial carcinoma of the bladder (SCB), stage PTa and GI (7 patients), GII (8 patients), GIII (3 patients). (B) 14 patients in follow-up for previous SCB and with negative cystoscopy and multiple bladder biopsies (MBB). (C) Control group: 21 with benign prostatic hypertrophy (BPH).

Cytology specimens were spun down in a Shandon Cytospin 2 centrifuge and stained according to the standard Papanicolau procedure. BW for flow cytometry were analyzed with an Epics Profile II (Coulter Co.). Briefly, this involves centrifugation at 1,500 rpm for 5 min and discarding the supernatant. The cell pellet is then resuspended in 3 ml cold phosphate-buffered saline with 7 ml. Cold 95% ethanol is added during vortexing. After centrifugation the pellets are stained with 5 ml propidium iodide staining solution and 0.1 mg/ml ribonuclease B. Each specimen is filtered through 37 nm nylon mesh before flow cytometry analysis. The specimens were interpreted as positive for cancer when there was an aneuploid stemline and/or when 15% or more of the measured cells showed hyperdiploid DNA (that is greater than 2c DNA content). A specimen was considered negative for cancer if no DNA aneuploid stemline could be detected and if fewer than 11% of the cells measured by bladder wash flow cytometry were hyperdiploid [11, 14, 15].

## Results

*BW Cytology*

*Group A:* In 16 patients with TCC, we obtained 10 BW with a positive cytological report for tumor (there being 2 GI, 5 GII and 3 GIII), one doubtful which was a GI and 5 false-negatives (normal cytology), the histological report of which was 4 GI and 1 GII TCC.

*Group B:* In 14 SCB control patients (with cystoscopy and MBB negative for TCC or carcinoma in situ, 9 BW reported as normal, 2 doubtful and 3 false-positives (1 of them with moderate dysplasia in MBB).

Group control: In the 21 BPH, all cytology results were normal.

*BW Flow Cytometry*

*Group A:* In the group of SCB, we found 3 aneuploid histograms (there being 1 GII and 2 GIII TCC) and 7 cases of hyperdiploidy (over 16% of cells), there being 2 GI, 4 GII and 1 GIII TCC. The mean proliferation index (PI) was 31% (between 20 and 44%). In the remainder of tumors the result of the histogram was euploid (5 GI and 1 GII TCC) with a proliferation index of 12% (between 4 and 26).

*Groups B and C:* In the groups of BPH and control with a clinical history of SCB, all histograms were normal, except for one false-positive hyperdiploid (over 16% in GII + M) in group C. The overall mean PI was 14% (between 7 and 31%).

## Discussion

Most authors give a higher diagnostic sensitivity to flow cytometry in SBC over classical or wash cytology [14–16]. The better diagnostic performance of wash cytology over classical cytology has also been demonstrated [5, 16]. Flow cytometry reaches a diagnostic sensitivity of 80–85% in the SCB, with only 5% of false-positives, following the criteria of Collste et al. [9]: existence of aneuploidy and/or over 15% of hyperdiploid cells. In this line, only 7% of SCB GI are diagnosed. Some authors have achieved 91% with other criteria [11], but at the cost of 30% false-positives. The role of wash cytology and flow cytometry being added to the diagnosis of SCB is debatable [1].

In our series we found a perfect correlation between both, with a diagnostic sensitivity of 63% (10/16), although flow cytometry only had 2.9% false-positives (1/35) compared with 14% (5/35) from BW cytology. These results are in line with what has been found by other authors [17–19], albeit with diagnostic indices close to 75%. Diagnosis by degrees of tumor was the same as the two procedures, not improving with its addition: 2 out of 7 GI (both hyperdiploid), 5 out of 6 GII (1 aneuploid and 4 hyperdiploid) and 3 out of 3 GIII TCC (2 aneuploid and 1 hyperdiploid).

*To conclude:* flow cytometry and BW cytology have been shown to be highly sensitive for diagnosing degrees II–III TCC, but very little in GIs. Flow cytometry did not significantly improve the diagnostic information of BW cytology.

## References


1 Badalament RA, Hermansen DK, Kimmel M, Gay H, Herr HW, Fair WR, Whitmore WF, Melamed M: The sensitivity of bladder wash flow cytometry, bladder wash cytology, and voided cytology in the detection of bladder carcinoma. Cancer 1987;60:1423–1427.

2 Cowan D, Wu B, Young G, Khanna P: Correlation of histopathological, cytological and flow cytometric findings in neoplasic and nonneoplasic lesions of the bladder. J Urol 1987;138:753–757.

3 Boileau M, Swartz D, Schmidt K, Schmidt W: Limitations of flow cytometric DNA analysis for the diagnosis of bladder cancer. J Surg Oncol 1989;40:194–200.

4 Colpeaert C, Goovaerts G, Buyssens N: Factors influencing the subjective grading of bladder cancer. Virchows Arch [A] 1987;411:479–484.

5 Pauwels R, Smeets A, Schapers R, Beck H: Are cytoflowmetry or chromosome studies or other predictors of any help determining the prognosis of low-grade superficial tumors? Th Pr Urol Cancer 1989;61:503–510.

6 Abel P, Henderson D, Bennett M, Hall R, Williams G: Differing interpretations by pathologists of the pT category and grade of transitional cell cancer of the bladder. Br J Urol 1988;62:339–342.

7 Lutzeyer W, Rubben H, Dahm H: prognostic parameter in superficial bladder cancer: An analysis of 315 cases. J Urol 1982;127:250–252.

8 Deitch A, Strand M, deVere White R: Flow cytometry: Developing role in the management of urologic disease; in deVere White W (ed): New Techniques in Urology. New York, futura Publishing Co, 1987, chapt 10, pp 137–159.

9 Collste L, Devonec M, Darzynkiewicz Z, et al: Bladder cancer diagnosis by flow cytometry. Correlation between cell samples from biopsy and bladder irrigation fluid. Cancer 1980;45:2389.

10 Bretton P, Myc A, Cordon C, DeAngelis P, Fair W, Melamed M: Initital evaluation of new epithelial antigen (T16) for bivariate flow cytometry of bladder irrigation specimens. Cytometry 1989;10:339–344.

11 Klein FA, Herr H, Sogani P, Withmore W, Melamed M: Flow cytometry of normal and nonneoplastic diseases of the bladder: an estimate of false-positive rate. J Urol 1982;127:946–948.

12 Jitsukawa S, Tachibana M, Nakazono M, Zazaki H, Addonizio J: Flow cytometry based on heterogeneity index score compared with urine cytology to evaluate their diagnostic efficacy in bladder tumor. Urology 1987;29:218–222.

13 Malstrom P, Vasko J, Wester K, Norlen B, Busch C: Flow cytometric analysis of DNA content of deparaffinized nuclei in urinary bladder carcinomas. APMIS 1989;97:811–819.

14 Hermansen D, Badalament R, Fair W, Kimmel M, Whitmore W, Melamed M: Detection of bladder carcinoma in females by flow cytometry and cytology. Cytometry 1989;10:739–742.

15 Lipponen P, Eskelinen M, Collan Y, Pesonen E, Ventila T, Sotarauta M, Norling S: DNA ploidy and S-phase fraction in human bladder cancer. Urol Int 1990;45:4–9.

16 Smeets A, Pauwels R, Beck H, Feitz W, Geraeds J, Debruyne F, Laaeakkers L, Vooijs G, Ramaeckers F: Comaprison of tissue disaggregation techniques of transitional cell bladder carcinomas for flow cytometry and chromosomal analysis. Cytometry 1987;8:14–19.

17 Klein FA, White FK: Flow cytometry deoxyribonucleic acid determinations and cytology of bladder washings: practical experience. J Urol 1988;139:275–278.

18 Blomjous E, Nellie W, Schipper P, Baak J, Winand V, DeVoogt H, Meijer C: The value of morphometry and DNA flow cytometry in addition to classic prognosticators in superficial urinary bladder carcinoma. AJCP 1989;91:243–248.

19 Konchuba A, Schellhammer P, Alexander J, Wright G: Flow cytometric study comparing paired bladder washing and voided urine for bladder cancer detection. Urology 1989;33:89–96.

Eur Urol 1992;21(suppl 1):16–21

M.C. Sanchez-Fernandez de Sevilla[a]
M. Gil-Salom[b]
M. Perez-Bacete[a]
L. Morell-Quadreny[a]
F. Martinez-Diaz[a]
I. Iborra-Juan[c]
B. Fenollosa-Entrena[d]
A. Llombart-Bosch[a]

# DNA-Ploidy, Morphometric-Stereological and P-Glycoprotein Study of Superficial Bladder Carcinomas

[a] Department of Pathology (Prof. *A. Llombart Bosch)* and
[b] Service of Urology (Department of Surgery), University of Valencia;
[c] Instituto Valenciano de Oncologia, Valencia, and
[d] Preventive Medicine Service, La Fe Hospital, Valencia, Spain

**Key Words**
Bladder cancer
DNA
Morphometry
Stereology
P-glycoprotein

**Abstract**
We carried out a DNA-ploidy, morphometric-stereologic and P-glycoprotein study on 40 newly diagnosed superficial bladder cancer patients (G1-G2), correlating the results with histological grade and clinical outcome. Variations in the number of patients who present recurrences, progression or remain tumor-free during the whole follow-up period (at least 5 years) were not significant when related to nuclear size, proliferative diploid index, presence of aneuploidy and expression of P-glycoprotein. It is striking how the majority of disease-free subjects showed a proliferative diploid index higher than 10%. Moreover, 3 of them presented an aneuploid cell population. In our study, only histological grade showed a significant discriminatory level in terms of progression versus no progression in patients with superficial bladder cancer.

## Introduction

One of the primary aims in bladder transitional cell carcinomas is to predict the prognosis in patients with low-grade (G1-G2), low-stage (Ta-T1) tumors [1]. It is well known that, at presentation, 70–75% of patients with bladder cancer have superficial tumors, that 70% of them will recur, and that 10–15% of recurrences will be invasive carcinomas. The remaining 25–30% of patients with bladder cancer have already at presentation invasive tumors [2].

The aim of the present study was to detect, among the patients with superficial tumors, the group with 'high risk' to progress to invasive carcinomas. Therefore, we evaluated 40 newly diagnosed patients with superficial bladder cancer by means of a DNA-ploidy, morphometric-stereologic and P-glycoprotein study, correlating the results with histological grade and clinical outcome (recurrence, progression and 5-year disease-free survival).

## Materials and Methods

TUR specimens from 40 newly diagnosed superficial bladder cancer patients (37 males, 3 females, mean age 67) were studied. No patient had been treated previously with chemotherapy or radiotherapy. Tumor grade and stage was established according to Mostofi's [3] and UICC [4] systems.

The most representative tumor areas were selected and photographed for morphometric study. Both superficial and basal zones of tumor papillae were separately evaluated, counting at least 300 nuclei per tumor. Black and white photographs were performed with

Carmen Sanchez-Fernandez de Sevilla, MD
Department of Pathology, University of Valencia
Av. Blasco Ibanez, 17
E-46010 Valencia (Spain)


0302–2838/92/0215–0016
$2.75/0

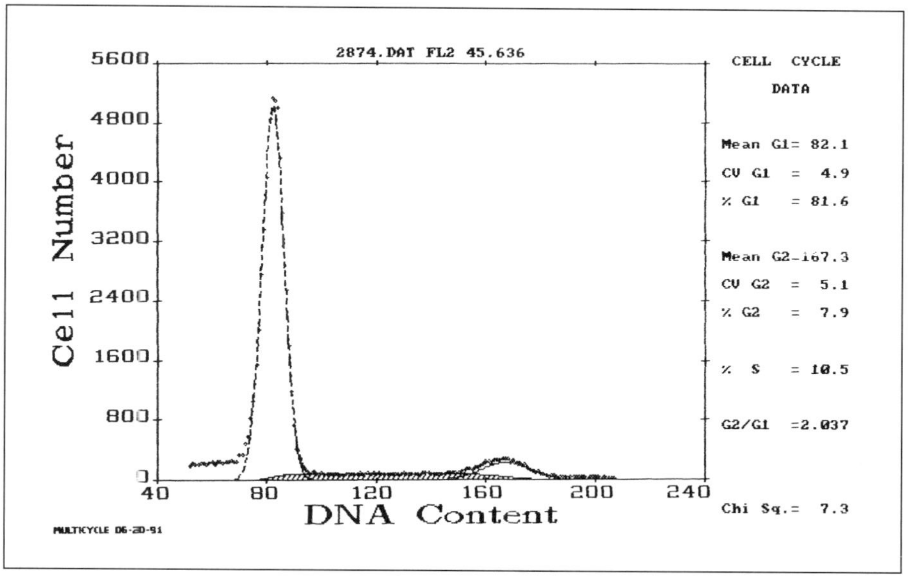


**Fig. 1.** DNA histogram of a bladder tumor with diploid cell population.

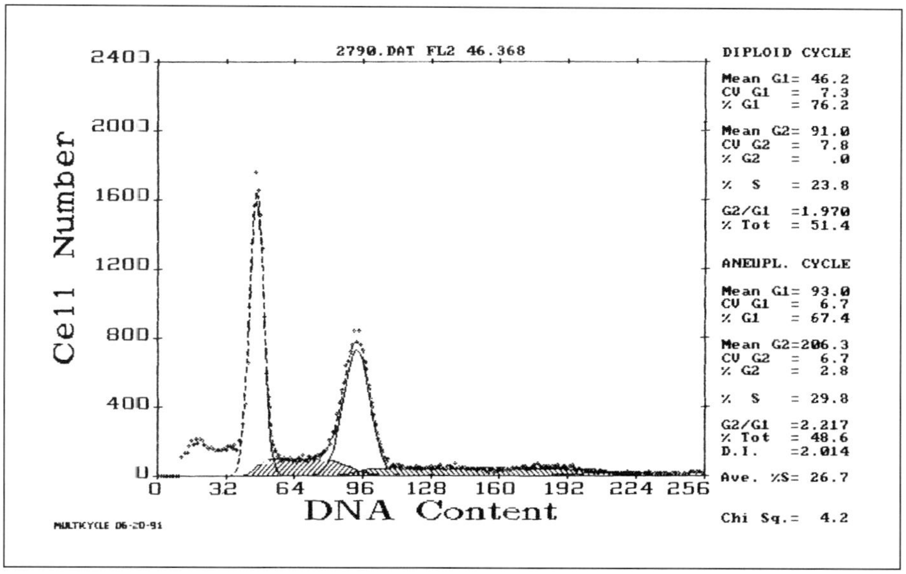


**Fig. 2.** DNA histogram of a bladder tumor with diploid and triploid cell populations.

a photomicroscope (Nikon) at 40 × and were amplified to 1,000 × standard. Measures were obtained with a semiautomatic image-analysis system (MOP Videoplan 2000, Zeiss Kontron). Nuclear area, nuclear perimeter and nuclear maximum diameter were selected as most representative morphometric parameters, and a shape-factor related to nuclear sphericity, nuclear volumetric density and nuclear numerical density were selected as stereologic parameters.

DNA-ploidy values were obtained from 40–μm thick, paraffin-embedded tissue sections, from which the nuclei were extracted using Hedley's tissue separation method. At least 10,000 nuclei per tumor were processed using a Coulter-Profile analyzer. The presence of diploid (fig. 1) and aneuploid (triploid (fig. 2) or tetraploid (fig. 3)) populations and their proliferative index (PI = S + G2/M) were recorded.

P-glycoprotein (multidrug resistance protein) expression was studied with the avidin-biotin (ABC) system, using diaminobenzidine as revealer and the antibodies C-219 (Centocor) and JB-1 (Monosan, Sambio).

Intravesical instillations of adriamycin was the only post-TUR treatment in each patient. Patients were followed up at least for 5 years, with cystoscopies and urinary cytologies. According to their clinical outcome, patients were classified in three groups: tumor-free (those with no recurrences or progression), recurrences (those with one or more recurrences during the follow-up period, but always low-grade, low-stage), and progression (those who progressed to invasive or metastatic bladder carcinoma).

For statistical evaluation $\chi^2$ test and paired and unpaired t tests (with Yates correction when required) were used.

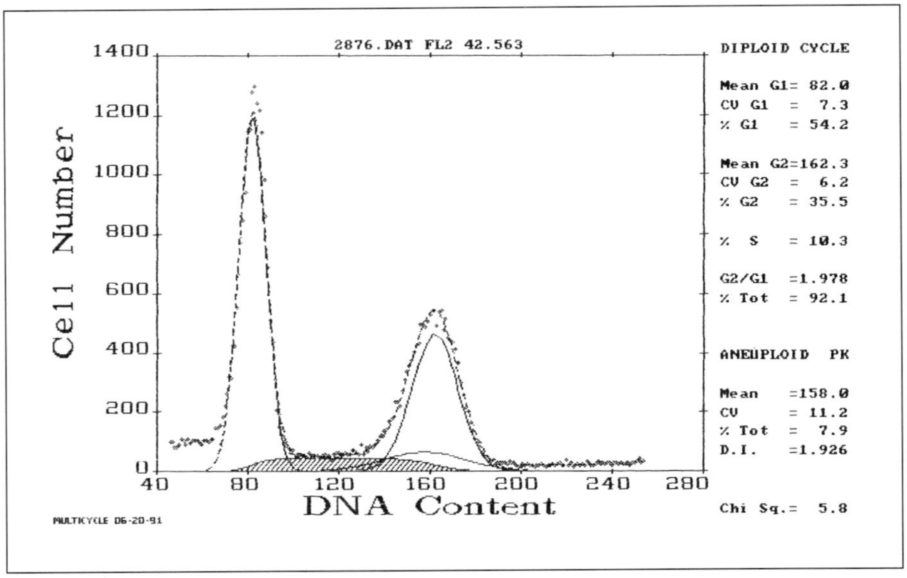


**Fig. 3.** DNA histogram of a bladder tumor with diploid and tetraploid cell populations.

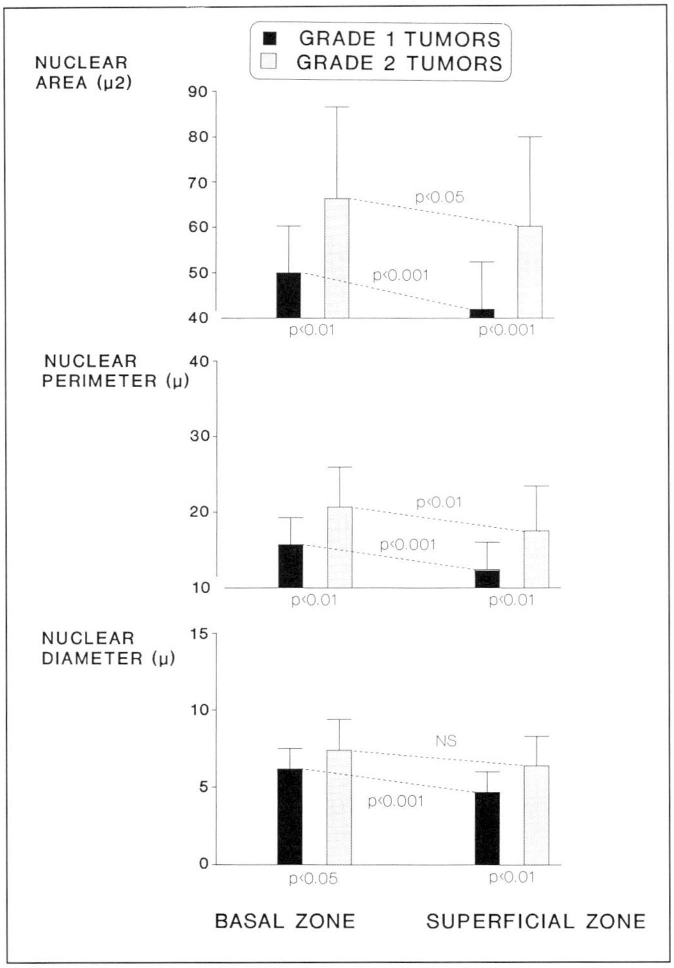


**Fig. 4.** Correlation between morphometry and tumor grade. NS: not significant ( t test).

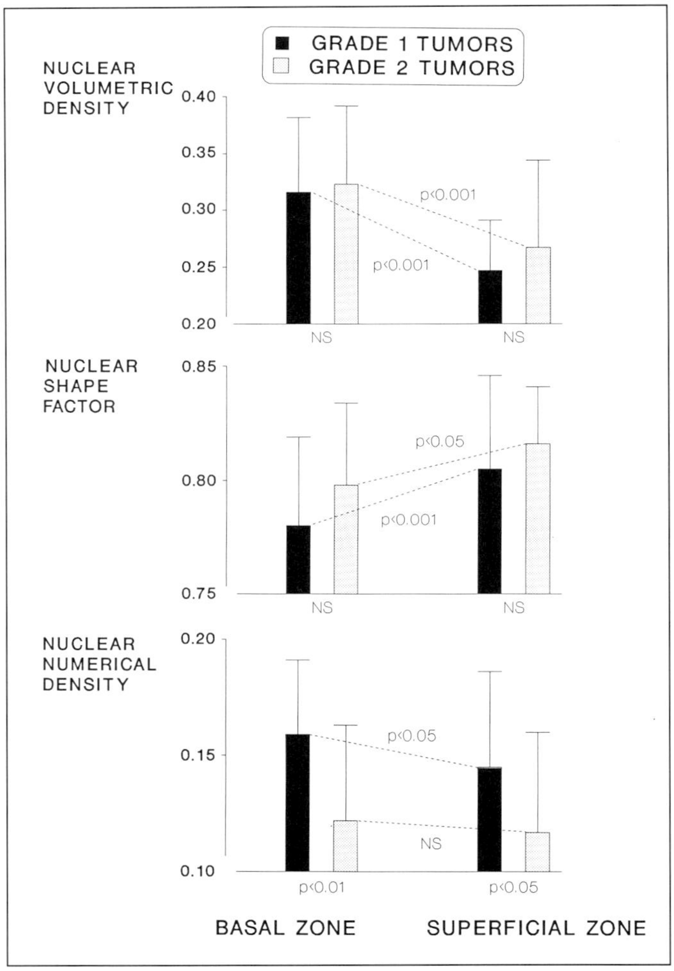


**Fig. 5.** Correlation between stereology and tumor grade. NS: not significant (t test).

## Results

Twenty-three tumors were G1 and 17 were G2. Thirty-nine tumors were suitable for morphometric and stereological study. Morphometry of superficial and basal zones of G1 tumors showed significant differences for nuclear area, perimeter and diameter. Such differences were also seen in G2 tumors, but of less statistical significance. A higher standard deviation of values in G2 tumors (reflecting more anisokaryosis) than in G1 tumors was evident (fig. 4).

Stereology showed significant differences only when studying nuclear numerical density, with higher values (more nuclei per volume unit, but smaller) in G1 than in G2 tumors (fig. 5).

Thirty-five tumors were suitable for DNA-ploidy study. Number of patients with diploid and aneuploid cell populations according to tumor grade are shown in table 1. Most tumors with PI < 10% were G1, while most aneuploid tumors were G2. Thirty-one tumors were suitable for P-glycoprotein study, 21 being positive (13 G1, 8 G2) and 10 negative (7 G1, 3 G2). When comparing these results with clinical outcome (table 2), only tumor grade determined significant differences ($p < 0.05$) between patients who progressed and those who did not (free of disease or with low-grade, low-stage recurrences).

**Table 1.** DNA-ploidy related to tumor grade

| | G1 tumors | G2 tumors |
|---|---|---|
| Diploid index <10% | 4 | 1 |
| Diploid index >10% | 17 | 13 |
| Aneuploid index | 2 | 4 |

**Table 2.** Correlation of parameters studied with clinical outcome

| | Tumor-free | Recurrences | Progression |
|---|---|---|---|
| Tumor grade (n = 40) | | | |
| Grade 1 | 13 | 8 | 2 |
| Grade 2 | 6 | 4 | 7 |
| Nuclear area (n = 39) | | | |
| $< 55\ \mu m^2$ | 11 | 10 | 1 |
| $> 55\ \mu m^2$ | 7 | 6 | 4 |
| Diploid index (n = 35) | | | |
| <10% | 2 | 2 | 1 |
| >10% | 14 | 10 | 6 |
| Aneuploid index (n = 35) | | | |
| Yes | 3 | 1 | 2 |
| No | 13 | 11 | 5 |
| P-glycoprotein (n = 31) | | | |
| Positive | 10 | 7 | 4 |
| Negative | 5 | 4 | 1 |

Tumor-free + Recurrences vs. Progression according to tumor grade: $p < 0.05$ ($\chi^2$ test with Yates correction).

## Discussion

Clinical outcome of patients with superficial bladder cancer is difficult to predict. The variability of natural history of these tumors was stressed 35 years ago by Marshall [5], who reported that 5-year survival of patients with high-grade superficial tumors was 50%, whereas of patients with low-grade superficial tumors varies widely between 37 and 71%. Multiple systems have been developed [3, 6–12], but grading criteria are variable and subjective. Moreover, some low-grade tumors progress to invasion and death, their malignant potential being underscored by grading systems.

Tumors stage (T1 vs. Ta) is considered as a more objective risk factor for recurrence and progression in superficial bladder cancer than is grade [13, 14]. However, the usefulness of staging systems [4] has been limited by the lack of accuracy in assessing the clinical extent of disease, with understaging errors around 25% [15–18].

Therefore, parameters other than grade and stage are needed for a better characterization of malignant potential and prognosis in low-grade superficial bladder cancer [1]. The prognostic value of tumor size, multiplicity and abnormalities in mucosal biopsies is well known [13, 14, 19–21]. In the last decade numerous studies have been carried out to search for new prognostic factors, already present at initial evaluation, which could be applied in clinical setting for adopting a more aggressive therapeutic attitude or a closer follow-up in patients with high risk to develop invasive tumors: cytogenetic studies [22–26], blood group isoantigens deletion [27–31], ultrastructural early neoplastic changes detection [32–35], immunologic studies [36–39], and those evaluated in the present work. Results of these studies have been variable, and sometimes very promising, but their clinical utility has to be proven by a more ample clinical experience.

Nuclear area has been found to correlate with tumor grade [40–42], and high area values have been reported to determine a poor prognosis [43–45]. In our study both morphometric and stereologic parameters showed significant differences when evaluating separately basal and superficial tumoral zones, thus reflecting the progressive cytodifferentiation from basal to superficial urothelial cells. Most of the parameters studied vary significantly according to tumor grade. Morphometric and stereological parameters did not, however, correlate with clinical outcome in our patients.

Aneuploid tumors have been reported to recur and progress more frequently than diploid ones, and the diploid proliferative index has also been considered as a prognostic factor [46–50]. In our study no significant correlations between DNA-ploidy and tumor grade were found. Among the patients who progressed most had a proliferative diploid index higher than 10%, but without reaching statistical significance. It is striking how the majority of disease-free subjects showed a proliferative diploid index higher than 10% and how 3 of them presented an aneuploid cell population. Thus, as stated by others [51, 52], ploidy as measured by DNA flow cytometric seems to be not sufficiently reliable in the prediction of disease progression to allow modification of therapy.

Expression of the multidrug resistance gene product (P-glycoprotein) [53, 54] was positive in 67% of patients free of disease, in 64% of patients who recur and in 75% of patients who progressed, these differences being not significant.

We therefore conclude that in our study, of all parameters evaluated, only histological grade, in spite of its limitations, showed a significant discriminatory level in terms of progression versus no progression in patients with superficial bladder cancer.

## References


1 Javadpour N: Multiple cell markers in bladder cancer: Principles and clinical applications. Urol Clin North Am 1984;11:609–616.

2 Lutzeyer W, Rubben H, Dahm H: Prognostic parameters in superficial bladder cancer: an analysis of 315 cases. J Urol 1982;127:250–252.

3 Mostofi FK: Histological typing of urinary bladder tumors; in International Histological Classification of Tumors. Geneva, WHO, 1973, vol 10.

4 Spiessl B, Beahrs O, Hermanek P, Hutter RVP, Scheibe O, Sobin LH, Wagner G: TNM Atlas, ed 3. Berlin, Springer, 1989, pp 245–250.

5 Marshall WF: Current clinical problems regarding bladder tumors. Cancer 1956;9:543–551.

6 Broders AC: Epithelioma of the genitourinary organs. Ann Surg 1922;75:574–604.

7 Asch JE: Epithelial tumors of the bladder. J Urol 1940;44:135–141.

8 Franksson C: Tumors of the bladder. J Urol 1940;44:135–141.

9 Bergkvist A, Ljunquist A, Moberger G: Classification of bladder tumors based on the cellular pattern. Preliminary report of a clinical pathological study of 300 cases with a minimum follow-up of eight years. Acta Chir Scand 1965; 130:371–378.

10 Pugh RC: The pathology of cancer of the bladder. Cancer 1973;32:1267–1274.

11 Friedell GH, Bell JR, Burney SW, Soto EA, Tiltman AJ: Histopathology and classification of urinary bladder carcinoma. Urol Clin North Am 1976;3:53–70.

12 Prout GR: Classification and staging of the bladder carcinoma. Cancer 1980;45:1832–1841.

13 Heney NM, Nocks NM, Daly JJ, Prout GR, Newall JB, Griffin PB, Perrone TL, Szyfelbein WA: Ta and T1 bladder cancer: Location recurrence and progression. Br J Urol 1982;54:152–157.

14 Heney NM, Ahmed S, Flanagan MJ, Frable W, Corder MP, Hafermann MD, Hawkins IR: Superficial bladder cancer: progression and recurrence. J Urol 1983;130:1083–1086.

15 Marshall WF: The relation of the preoperative estimate to the pathologic demonstration of the extent of vesical neoplasms. J Urol 1952;68: 714–723.

16 Schmidt JD, Weinstein SH: Pitfalls in clinical staging of bladder tumours. Urol Clin North Am 1976;3:107–127.

17 Kenny GM, Hardner GJ, Murphy GP: Clinical staging of bladder tumours. J Urol 1970;104: 720–723.

18 Prout GR: The surgical management of bladder carcinoma. Urol Clin North Am 1976;3: 149–153.

19 Eisenberg RB, Roth RB, Schweinsberg RH: Bladder tumors and associated proliferative mucosal lesions. J Urol 1960;84:544–550.

20 Schade ROK, Swinney J: The association of urothelial abnormalities with neoplasia: a 10-year follow-up. J Urol 1983;129:1125–1126.

21 Althausen AF, Prout GR, Daly JJ: Non-invasive papillary carcinoma of bladder associated with carcinoma in situ. J Urol 1976;116:576–579.

22 Falor WH, Ward RH: Prognosis in early carcinoma of the bladder based on chromosomal analysis. J Urol 1978;119:44–48.

23 Spooner ME, Cooper EH: Chromosome constitution of transitional cell carcinoma of the urinary bladder. Cancer 1972;29:1401–1412.

24 Cummings KB: Carcinoma of the bladder: Predictors. Cancer 1980;45:1849–1855.

25 Summers JL, Falor WH, Ward R: A 10-year analysis of chromosomes in non-invasive papillary carcinoma of the bladder. J Urol 1981;125:177–178.

26 Sandberg AA: Chromosome markers and progression in bladder cancer. Cancer Res 1977; 37:2950–2956.

27 Decenzo JM, Howard P, Irish CE: Antigenic detection A, B, H and prognosis of patients with stage A transitional cell bladder carcinoma. J Urol 1975;114:874–878.

28 Newman AJ, Carlton CE, Johnson S: Cell surface A, B, or O(H) blood group antigens as an indicator of malignant potential in bladder carcinoma. J Urol 1980;124:27–29.

29 Catalona WJ: Practical utility of specific red cell adherence test in bladder cancer. Urology 1981;18:113–117.

30 Stein BS, Reyes J, Petersen RO, McNellis D, Kendall AR: Specific red cell adherence, immunologic evaluation of random mucosal biopsies in carcinoma of the bladder. J Urol 1981;126:37–42.

31 Weinstein RS, Coon J, Alroy J, Davidson I: Tissue-associated blood group antigens in human tumors; in DeLellis RA (ed): Diagnostic Immunochemistry. New York, Masson, 1981, pp 239–261.

32 Hicks RM: Discussion on morphological markers of early neoplastic change in the urinary bladder. Cancer Res 1977;37:2822–2823.

33 Kahan BD, Rutzky LP, Kahan AV, Oyasu R, Wisehan F, Legrves S: Cell surface changes associated with malignant transformation of bladder epithelium in vitro. Cancer Res 1977; 37:2866–2871.

34 Koss LG: Some ultrastructural aspects of experimental and human carcinomas of the bladder. Cancer Res 1977;37:2824–2835.
35 Tannenbaum M: Conformational membrane changes in early bladder cancer; in Connolly JG (ed): Carcinoma of the Bladder. Progress in Cancer Research and Therapy. New York, Raven Press, 1981, vol 18, pp 115–126.
36 Catalona WJ, Chretien PB: Correlation among host immunocompetence and tumor stage, tumor grade and vascular permeation in transitional carcinoma. J Urol 1973;110:526–528.
37 Brosman S, Elhilali M, Vescera C, Fahey J: Immune response in bladder cancer patients. J Urol 1979;121:162–169.
38 Britten V, Rees RC, Clegg A, Smith GT, Potter CW, Fox M, Williams JL: Natural killer cell activity and response to phytohemagglutinin compared with the histological diagnosis of patients with transitional cell carcinoma of the bladder. Br J Urol 1982;54:261–266.
39 Gozzo JJ, Cronin WJ, O'Brien P, Monaco AP: Detection of tumor associated antigens in urine from patients with bladder cancer. J Urol 1980; 124:804–807.
40 Ooms EC, Kurver PH, Velduizen RW, Alons CL, Boon ME: Morphometric grading of bladder tumors in comparison with histologic grading by pathologists. Hum Pathol 1983;14:144–150.
41 Montironi R, Scarpelli M, Pisani E, Ansuini G, Mariuzzi GM: Histomorphometry and pattern recognition analysis of urothelial papillary lesions. Tumori 1984;70:463–466.
42 Helander K, Hofer P, Holmberg G: Karyometric investigations on urinary bladder carcinoma, correlated to histopathological grading. Virchows Arch [A] 1984;403:117–125.
43 Ooms EC, Essed E, Velduizen RW, Alons CL, Kurver P, Boon ME: The prognostic significance of morphometry in T1 bladder tumours. Histopathology 1981;5:311–318.
44 Boon ME, Kurver PHJ, Baak JPA, Ooms ECM: Morphometric differences between urothelial cells in voided urine of patients with grade I and grade II bladder tumours. J Clin Pathol 1981;34:612–615.
45 Boon ME, Baak JPA: Bladder: selection of patients with papillary T1 tumours with poor prognosis; in Baak JPA, Oort J (eds): Manual of Morphometry in Diagnostic Pathology. Berlin, Springer, 1983, pp 74–76.
46 Devonec H, Darzynkiewicz Z, Whitmore WF, Melamed MR: Flow cytometry for follow-up examinations of conservational treated low stage bladder tumors. J Urol 1981;126:166–170.
47 Gustafson H, Tribukait B, Esposti PL: DNA profile and tumor progression in patients with superficial bladder tumors. Urol Res 1982;10: 13–20.
48 Tribukait B, Gustafson H, Esposti PL: The signification of ploidy and proliferation in the clinical and biological evaluation of bladder tumours: A study of 100 untreated cases. Br J Urol 1982,45:130–135.
49 Oljans PJ, Tanke HJ: Flow cytometric analysis of DNA content in bladder cancer: prognostic value of the DNA index with respect to early tumour recurrence in G2 tumours. World J Urol 1986;4:205–210.
50 de Vere White R, Deitel AD, West B, Fitzpatrick JM: The predictive value of flow cytometric information in the clinical management of stage 0 (Ta) bladder cancer. J Urol 1988;139: 279–282.
51 Brendler ChB: Flow cytometric evaluation of urological malignancy. Editorial. J Urol 1988; 139:342–343.
52 Pauwels R, Smeets A, Schapers R, Beck H: Are cytoflowmetry or chromosome studies or other predictors of any help determining the prognosis of low-grade superficial tumors? In Murphy G, Khoury S (eds): Therapeutic Progress in Urological Cancers. New York, Liss, 1989, pp 503–510.
53 Cordon-Cardo C, O'Brien JP, Boccia J, Casals D, Bertino JR, Melamed MR: Expression of the multidrug resistance gene product (P-glycoprotein) in human normal and tumor tissues. J Histochem Cytochem 1990;38:1277–1287.
54 Weinstein RS, Kuszak JR, Kluskens LF, Coon JS: The multidrug resistance gene family in humans. Hum Pathol 1990;21:34–48.

Eur Urol 1992;21(suppl 1):22–25

F. Di Silverio[a], M. von Heland[a]
E. De Berardinis[a], R. Izzi[a]
M. Buscarini[a], R. De Vita[b]
R. Forte[b], F. Seccareccia[c]
A. Menotti[c]

[a] Department of Urology, University 'La Sapienza';
[b] Environmental Biomedicine Division ENEA Casaccia, and
[c] Istituto Superiore di Sanità, Rome, Italy

# Prognostic Role of Flow Cytometry in Superficial Bladder Cancer

**Key Words**
Superficial bladder
Cancer-flow cytometry
Recurrences and/or progressions
Risk patient

**Abstract**
Prognostic factors in superficial transitional cell carcinoma of the bladder were assessed with histopathological and flow cytometry analysis in a series of 61 patients operated transurethrally between 1988 and 1990. In particular, we evaluated the usefulness of flow cytometry in order to identify patients who require a more accurate clinical follow-up or a more aggressive therapy. A multivariate analysis was done in 61 cases, considering patient age and sex, stage, grade and number of lesions (unifocal or multifocal), post-TUR therapy (therapy or not), and DNA ploidy (diploid/aneuploid). DNA pattern and number of recurrences were determinant for selecting risk cases for progression.

## Introduction

The incidence of transitional cell carcinoma of the bladder has steadily increased over the past 10 years. Bladder cancers now account for 3% of all cancer deaths in Italy while only for 1% in 1975. Superficial neoplasms make up 70% of all bladder cancers at the diagnosis; once the diagnosis is established they undergo transurethral endoscopic resection of the bladder. After the resection the problem of recurrence arises. There are several reports in the literature that indicate a 'new growth' frequency of 50–70% during the first 1–2 years. The 15% of recurrences will be an invasive carcinoma. A long-lasting clinical observation is therefore required in order to prevent the occurrence of 'new growths' or progressions. This implies a high-cost managing of the patient and a considerable amount of trouble for the patient himself who must frequently undergo invasive diagnostic procedures like cystoscopy. The purpose of this work has been trying to find one or more markers which could help us to discriminate the 'risk patient' from the 'nonrisk patient'. In fact, once the selection is made, it is possible to focalize clinical attention towards the first group of patients, leaving the others to live a less troubled life.

Magnus von Heland, MD
Department of Urology, University La Sapienza
Viale Del Policlinico Umberto I
I-00161 Rome (Italy)


0302–2838/92/0215–0022
$2.75/0

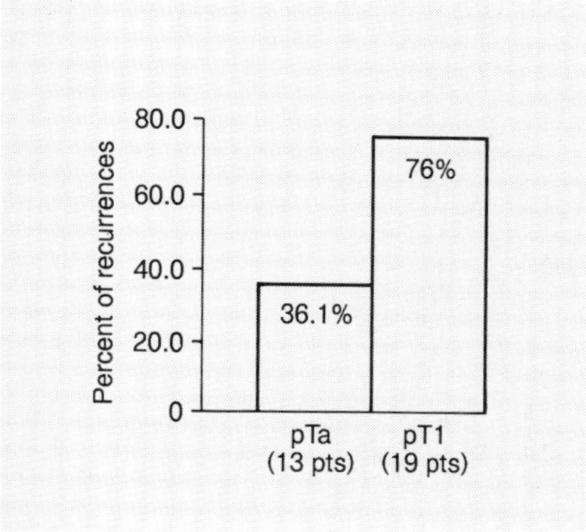


**Fig. 1.** Relation stage/recurrences. 32 recurrences/61 patients = 52.5%.

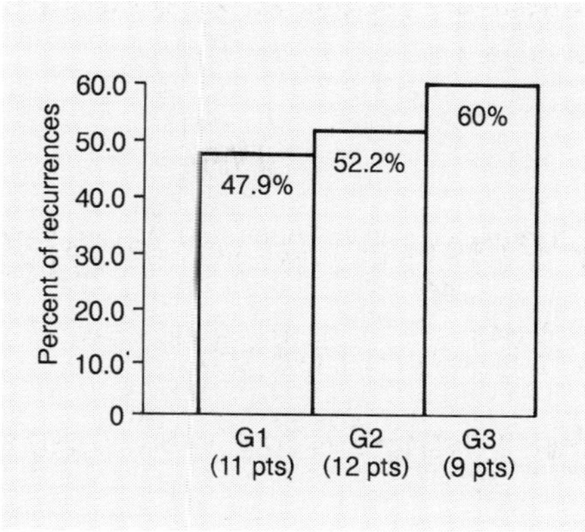


**Fig. 2.** Relation grade/recurrences. 32 recurrences/61 patients = 52.5%.

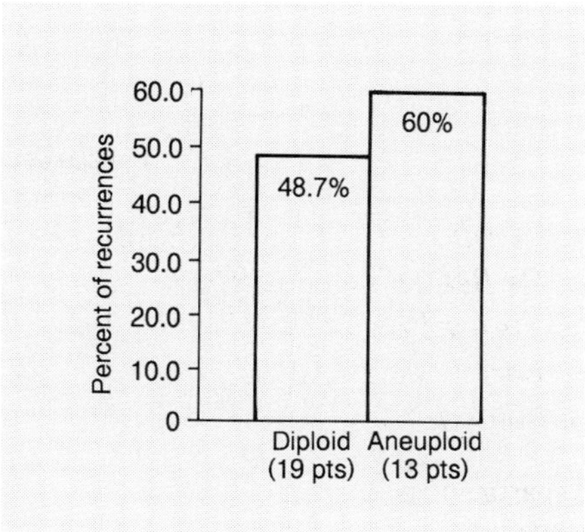


**Fig. 3.** Relation DNA/recurrences. 32 recurrences/61 patients = 52.5%.

## Material and Methods

Between 1988 and 1991, 61 patients (42 males, 19 females; age range 45–60) underwent TURB for superficial transitional cell carcinoma of the bladder. Their clinical follow-up (1 year minimum) was made up by echographical and cytological trials and cystoscopic examination every 6 months. If either urinary cytology or vesical echo were uncertain, cystoscopy was performed. Each recurrence brought us back to a new classification of the patient by means of TUR to assess staging, grading and ploidy of the neoplasms.

*Diagnostic Procedures*

Echographical evaluation was obtained through suprapubic scans (transverse and oblique) using a Brüel Kjaer 1846 instrument. Urinary cytology was performed by the same pathologist on three different specimens for each patient stained with 50% alcohol solution. For cystoscopy we eventually used Storz endoscopic instruments 17 and 19 Ch, equipped with 30, 70 and 120° optics.

*Study of Nuclear DNA Ploidy*

Flow cytometry was performed in the Laboratory of Dosimetry and Biophysics of ENEA. The samples were analyzed with a PAS II flow cytometer (Parter, Arlesheim, Switzerland). The signals were collected on a Master 4000 multichannel analyzer (Laben, Milan, Italy) and accumulated in memory. The histograms were stored on a floppy disk and analyzed by an original software on a PC IBM-XT. Flow cytometric analysis was performed according to the literature. Briefly, for each case analyzed, lymphocytes or normal bladder cell sample of the same patient was used as an external and internal standard of cytometrically diploid DNA content. Samples exhibiting one subpopulation with an abnormal DNA center were defined as cytometrically aneuploid.

*Statistical Analysis*

A multivariate analysis of the prognostic factors was performed according to the Cox model and the multiple logistic function. The following covariates were assessed: patient age and sex; tumor stage; grade and number of lesions; DNA ploidy taking the probability to recur or progress as end-points. The evaluation was obtained by means of stepwise option using the maximum partial likelihood ratio method (MPLR). The assumed limit of significance to enter a term was 0.1 and the limit to remove a term 0.15.

## Results

During a period of 1 year, 32 recurrences were diagnosed; among these, 13 developed progression. In respect to the recurrence/staging ratio, only 13 (36%) of the 36 pTa developed a new growth; on the other hand, 19 of the 25 pT1 (76%) had a recurrence (fig. 1). We observed 47.9, 52.2 and 60% of recurrences in G1, G2 and G3 respectively (fig. 2). The recurrence/ploidy ratio showed 19 recurrences on 39 diploids (48.7%) and 13 recurrences on 22 aneuploids (60%) (fig. 3). If we analyze the progression/staging ratio it is possible to find that 3 Pta (24%) and 10 pT1 (52.6%) developed progression (fig. 4). Eventually progression/grading ratio indicates that there has been no progression in G1 while 50 and 78% are the chances of progression for G2 (12 recurrences) and G3 (9 recurrences), respectively (fig. 5). The difference in terms of progression rate between diploids and aneuploids is clear: only 11% of the diploids will develop progression, while 85% of aneuploids will experience it (fig. 6). Statistical evaluation (Cox and multiple logistic function) of recurrences and progressions indicates that neither patient's age and sex nor tumor's grade, stage, DNA ploidy and focality (mono or multi) can be taken as statistically valuable in order to predict recurrences (tables 1–3). Tumor ploidy, instead, is the only parameter that can play a

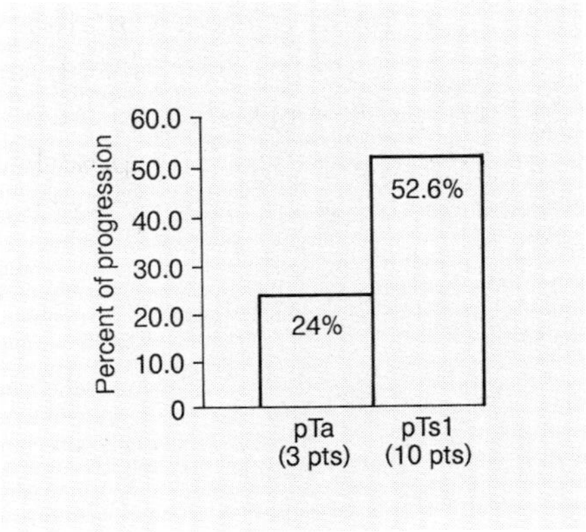


**Fig. 4.** Relation stage/progression (P). 13 P/32 recurrences = 40.6%.

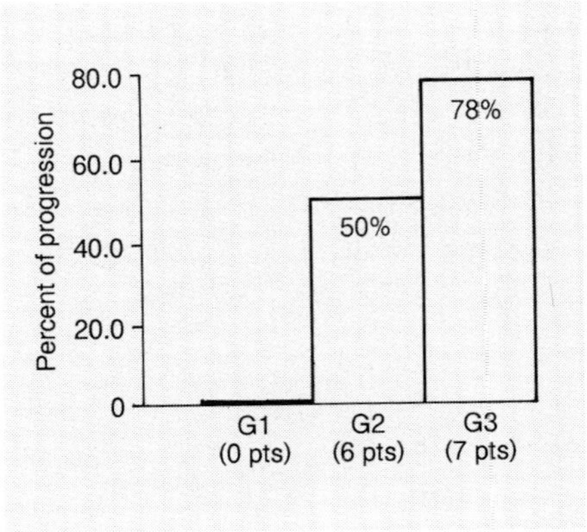


**Fig. 5.** Relation grade/progression (P). 13 P/32 recurrences = 40.6%.

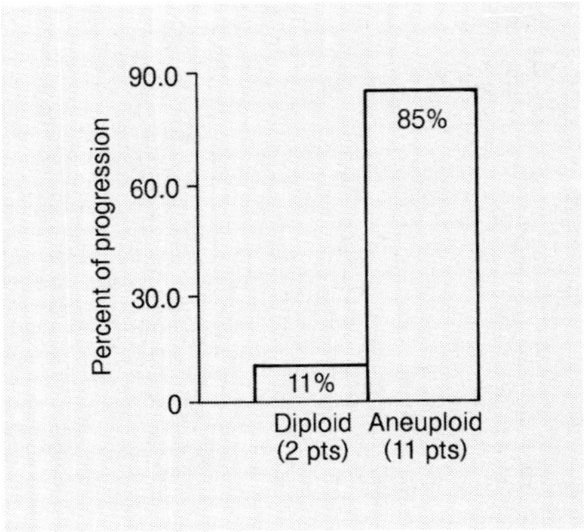


**Fig. 6.** Relation DNA/progression (P). 13 P/32 recurrences = 40.6%.

**Table 1.** Cox's hazard model

| Factor | Coefficient | t | p |
|---|---|---|---|
| Sex | 0.11174 | 0.1315 | NS |
| Age | −0.25844 | −0.6231 | NS |
| STGR | −0.31117 | −1.5040 | NS |
| DNA | 1.82440 | 2.0450 | <0.05 |
| Focality | 1.71880 | 1.4720 | NS |
| Constant | −3.10570 | −1.0300 | NS |

**Table 2.** Multiple logistic function (stepwise)

| Factor | Coefficient | t | p |
|---|---|---|---|
| DNA | 2.7460 | 2.090 | <0.05 |
| Focality | 1.8231 | 1.378 | NS |
| Constant | −7.7912 | −3.377 | NS |

**Table 3.** Multiple logistic function (stress)

| Factor | Coefficient | t | p |
|---|---|---|---|
| Sex | 0.6768 | 0.4295 | NS |
| Age | −0.0163 | −0.2481 | NS |
| STGR | −0.6950 | −1.7930 | NS |
| DNA | 3.0614 | 2.0670 | <0.05 |
| Focality | 2.0146 | 1.5630 | NS |
| Recurrence | 3.1066 | 2.8280 | <0.05 |
| Constant | −6.7056 | −1.3180 | NS |

major role in tumor's progression; in fact, either in Cox model or in multiple logistic function DNA evaluation showed a significant value referred to progressions.

## Conclusions

The results, according to our more extensive experience, indicate grade and stage invaluable as predictive criteria if taken separately. Conversely, combined use of these two tumor's characteristics shows that 42% of pT1 G3 progresses while only 4% of pTa G1 does. Stage and grade are still inadequate in intermediate cases (pTa–pT1 G2). For this reason we focalized our attention on flow cytometry and were able to demonstrate the latter being a valuable predictive parameter specially for the tumor's progression rate. Masters et al. [8] observed a pT1 progression rate of 4 and 35% among diploids and aneuploids respectively. Their results strictly resemble ours if we consider selected pT1 cases. The significance of tetraploid neoplasms still remains uncertain. Most authors group them together with diploid forms. Blomjous et al. [7] found that only patients with aneuploid superficial tumors developed progressive disease. This struggles with Murphy et al. [3] and De Vere White et al. [6] who observed that three quarters of Ta G1 and Ta G2 that became progressive were diploid.

In our study, 85% of the patients who developed recurrences with progression had aneuploid characteristics.

Comparing flow cytometry with urinary cytology some comments must be made: DNA ploidy studies require expensive equipment and trained technical support, but it seems that the diagnostic method is more trustworthy, reliable and repeatable than histopathological grading evaluation.

In conclusion, we emphasize that cellular DNA determination does not show any predictive significance for the tumor likelihood to recur, but seems instead to be a good marker related to the probability for a superficial bladder tumor to progress. That makes possible: (a) to select a 'non risk' group that will be followed up by means of noninvasive diagnostic technique; (b) to propose for the future a remarkable improvement of flow cytometry as far as cost and benefit are concerned.

## References


1 Heney NM, Ahmed S, Flanagan MJ, Frable W, Corder MP, Hafermann MD, Hawkins IR: Superficial bladder cancer: Progression and recurrence. National Bladder Cancer Collaborative Group. J Urol 1983;130:1083–1086.

2 Fossa SD, Kaalkus O: The prognostic relevance of nuclear Feulgen DNA in transitional cell carcinoma of the urinary bladder. Eur Urol 1985; 11:418–421.

3 Murphy WM, Chandler RW, Trafford RM: Flow cytometry of deparaffinated nuclei compared to histological grading for the pathological evaluation of transitional cell carcinomas. J Urol 1986;135:694–697.

4 Jakse G, Lodl W, Seeber G, et al: Stage T1 grade G3 transitional cell carcinoma of the bladder: An unfavorable tumor? J Urol 1987; 137:39–43.

5 Tribukait B: Flow cytometry in assessing the clinical aggressiveness of genitourinary neoplasms. World J Urol 1987;5:108.

6 De Vere White RW, Deitch AD, West B, Fitzpatrick JM: The predictive value of flow cytometry information in the clinical management of stage O (Ta) bladder cancer. J Urol 1988;139:279.

7 Blomjous CEM, Schipper NW, Baak JPA: Retrospective study of prognostic importance of DNA flow cytometry of urinary bladder carcinoma. J Clin Pathol 1988;41:21–25.

8 Masters JRW, Camplejohn RS, Parkinson MC, Woodhouse CRJ: DNA ploidy and the prognosis of stage Pt1 bladder cancer. Br J Urol 1989; 64:403–408.

9 De Vita R, Forte D, Maggi F, Eleuteri P, Di Silverio F: Cellular DNA content and proliferative activity evaluated by flow cytometry versus histopathological and staging classification in human bladder tumors. Eur Urol 1991;19: 65–73.

Eur Urol 1992;21(suppl 1):26–30

G.A. Saracino[a]
P. Ditonno[a]
G. Disabato[a]
A. Traficante[a]
M. Battaglia[a]
G. Lucivero[b]
F.P. Selvaggi[a]

[a] Department of Surgical Nephrology, University of Bari, and
[b] Department of Clinical Methodology, University of Napoli, Italy

# Prediction of Recurrence and Progression in Primary Superficial Bladder Cancer with DNA Flow Cytometry

**Key Words**
DNA flow cytometry
Bladder tumors
Intravesical prophylactic therapy

**Abstract**
Intravesical chemotherapy has been well established as an effective therapy for recurrent superficial bladder tumors. We investigated the role of flow cytometry as a predictor of tumor recurrence/progression after intravesical chemotherapy. Flow cytometric analysis of nuclear DNA ploidy pattern was performed on 'cold cup' biopsy samples of 52 patients with primary superficial bladder cancer. Cell suspensions, retrieved after mechanical fragmentation, were stained with propidium iodide and examined on FACScan flow cytometer. Clinical follow-up ranged from 3 to 57 months with a median of 20 months. Of the 52 patients, 24 aneuploid and 28 diploid tumors were observed. The degree of ploidy in relation to histological grade showed an increasing frequency of aneuploid pattern in grades 2 and 3 but with no statistical significance. 17.8% of diploid tumors versus 54.1% of aneuploid tumors recurred ($p < 0.05$). 12.5% of the aneuploid tumors progressed. No progression among diploid tumors was observed. Of the 52 patients examined, 35 (16 aneuploid and 19 diploid) were treated, after TUR, with intravesical prophylactic therapy. Epirubicin in 24, mitomycin C in 4 and recombinant interferon α2a in 7 were used. 50% of aneuploid tumors versus 10.5% of diploid tumors recurred ($p < 0.05$). Strong predictors of response to intravesical prophylaxis of recurrence were G1 grade and diploid DNA content.

## Introduction

Of superficial bladder cancers, nearly 70% recur and 10–20% progress within 2 years from the transurethral resection [1, 2]. The risk of progression is related to morphological and biological parameters such as grade, stage, tumor number and DNA flow cytometry [3–5]. Not all authors attributed the risk of recurrence to those parameters [2, 3, 5, 6]. In order to reduce the risk of progression/recurrence, several intravesical prophylactic regimens have been tested. This therapy, inefficient in 30–50% of cases [7–9], is expensive, requires good patient compliance and can have local and systemic side effects. To avoid this local chemotherapy in patients who do not recur and in those in whom the chemotherapy is ineffective, new biological parameters are tested. In this study,

Dr. Gabriele Alberto Saracino
Department of Surgical Nephrology
University of Bari
Piazzale Giulio Cesare, I-70124 Bari (Italy)


0302–2838/92/0215–0026
$2.75/0

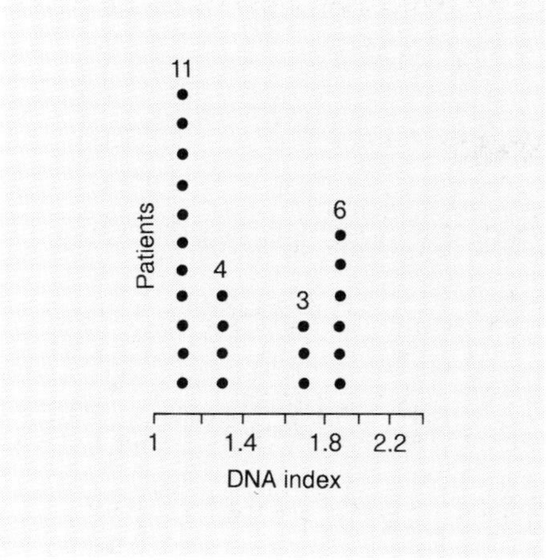


**Fig. 1.** The distribution of DNA index of aneuploid tumors is noncontinuous. The figure shows the absence of cellular population with DNA index between 1.4 and 1.6.

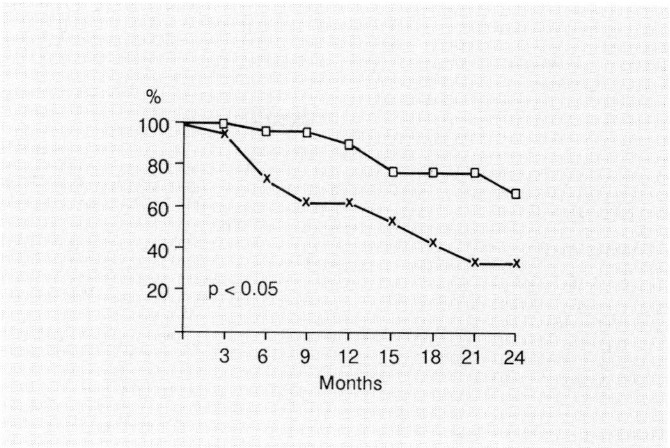


**Fig. 2.** Relationship between DNA content and recurrence. Mean follow-up is 20 months. Recurrence curves computed by log rank test. □ = Diploid tumors; × = aneuploid tumors.

we have investigated the value of DNA flow cytometry in assessing the risk of recurrence and progression in superficial bladder cancer. A comparative analysis with stage, grade and tumor number was also done.

## Materials and Methods

Fifty-two patients, 40 male and 12 female, with a mean age of 61 years (range 30–80), underwent transurethral resection of superficial bladder tumor between February 1986 and December 1990. Afterwards, 35 of 52 patients underwent intravesical prophylaxis: 24 were treated with epirubicin (Farmorubicina®; Farmitalia, Milano, Italy) (50 mg/50 ml of water, weekly 4 times, then monthly 11 times), 4 with mitomycin C® (Kiowa) (40 mg/40 ml of saline solution, weekly 8 times) and 7 with recombinant interferon-α2b (Intron A®; Schering Corp., Kenilworth, N.J., USA) (50 million IU/50 ml of saline solution, weekly 8 times).

The end-point of the study was the first recurrence and/or the progression to invasive cancer. Mean follow-up was 20 months (range 3–57). Tumors were classified according to the recommendation of the International Union Against Cancer and the World Health Organization.

Flow cytometric analysis of nuclear DNA ploidy pattern was performed on 'cold cup' biopsy samples. Cell suspensions, retrieved after mechanical fragmentation, were stained with a solution of Nonidet 0.1%, RNAse (Sigma, St. Louis, Mo., USA) 100 U/ml and propidium iodide (Sigma) 50 μg/ml and filtered with 35-μm filters. This stained cell population was examined on a FACScan flow cytometer (Becton Dickinson) with a 488-nm argon laser. An average of 10,000 cells were examined. The DNA values of analyzed cells were calculated with the DNA content of normal human lymphocytes (2c) as internal standard. The tumors were subdivided according to their DNA pattern into diploid (2c), tetraploid (4c) and aneuploid. A specimen was considered aneuploid when there was an additional distinct peak in the histogram, when the proportion of tetraploid cells exceeded 10%, when the histogram deviated more than 10% from the internal standard of normal lymphocytes or when the peak variation coefficient (CV) excceded 9%. In aneuploid specimens a ratio between the aneuploid and the diploid peak channels (DNA index) was calculated.

Statistical analysis was performed using the $\chi^2$ test, Kaplan-Meyer survival curves and the log rank test.

**Table 1.** Correlation between tumor grade and ploidy

| | G1 | G2 | G3 | Total |
|---|---|---|---|---|
| Diploid tumors | 17 | 9 | 2 | 28 |
| Aneuploid tumors | 9 | 11 | 4 | 24 |

## Results

### *Recurrence*

Of the 52 patients, 24 had aneuploid and 28 had diploid tumors. The degree of ploidy in relation to the histological grade showed an increasing frequency of the aneuploid pattern in grades 2 and 3 but with no statistical significance (table 1). The distribution of DNA index was noncontinuous and most of the tumors resulted near diploid (DNA index $<1.2$) and tetraploid (DNA index $>1.8$) (fig. 1). No tumors with a DNA index between 1.4 and 1.6 were observed. After a mean follow-up of 20 months (range 3–57), 5/28 diploid tumors (17.8%) and 13/24 aneuploid tumors (54.1%) recurred ($p < 0.05$) (fig. 2). Recurrence was evaluated in patients who re-

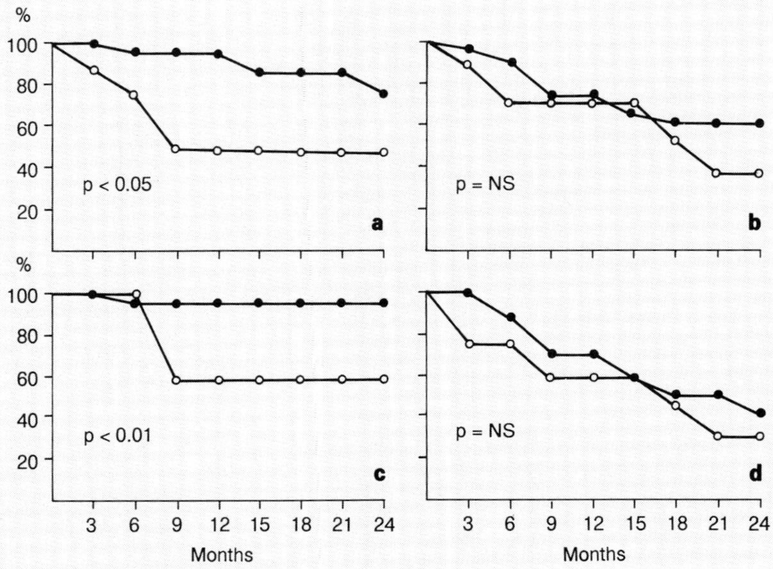


**Fig. 3.** Role of ploidy and tumor grade for prediction of recurrence in treated and untreated patients with prophylactic therapy. Recurrence curves computed by log rank test. **a** Diploid tumors; **b** aneuploid tumors; **c** grade 1 tumors; **d** grade 2–3 tumors. ● = Prophylaxis; ○ = no prophylaxis.

ceived prophylactic therapy and in untreated patients: 10 of the 35 patients of the treated group (28.5%) and 8 of 17 of the untreated group (47%) recurred ($p < 0.05$).

Separately, treated and untreated patients were stratified on the basis of ploidy, grade, stage and tumor number to assess the predictive value of these parameters for recurrence (table 2). Intravesical prophylaxis significantly reduced the recurrence rate in diploid and G1 tumors (fig. 3). We evaluated whether an additive predictive value could be observed when these parameters were associated. 17 tumors, 12 treated and 5 untreated, were G1 and diploid. Of these, only 1 patient, in the untreated group, recurred. This group of patients represents the one with the better prognosis for recurrence.

*Progression*

None of the diploid tumors and 3 of the aneuploid tumors (13%) progressed ($p < 0.05$). No difference in the progression rate between treated and untreated patients was observed (table 3). High-grade, T1 stage and multiplicity were associated parameters in the progressed tumors (table 4).

## Discussion

Our data confirmed a relationship between tumor stage and grade and DNA ploidy, as already shown in previous studies, although a statistical significance was not found due to the small number of cases. The noncontinuous DNA distribution was already reported by Devonec [10], who, on the base of this observation, hypothesized a 3-step theory for the progression of bladder tumors. The first step is the transforming event that causes a minimal change in cellular DNA content (diploid or near diploid cells); during the second step the cell undergoes chromosomal duplication whtout cell division becoming tetraploid; finally, in the third step, amounts of DNA are lost by the cell, which becomes aneuploid. For this reason, in superficial bladder cancer, which have not reached this third step, it is rare to find a DNA index in the range of 1.4 and 1.6.

In a clinical setting, DNA ploidy alone appears not to be sufficient to estimate the risk of recurrence. In our study, tumor recurrence was observed significantly less often in diploid tumors (17.8 vs. 54.1% of aneuploid tumors), but not enough to modify the standard follow-up program.

DNA ploidy appears to be reliable parameter to assess the risk of progression. In fact, our data showed no progression in the diploid tumors and a 12.5% progression

Table 2. Recurrence rate in relation to parameters of tumor

| | Prophylaxis | | | No prophylaxis | | | p |
|---|---|---|---|---|---|---|---|
| | pts | progr. | % | pts | progr. | % | |
| Diploid | 19 | 2 | 10.5 | 9 | 3 | 33.3 | < 0.05 |
| Aneuploid | 16 | 8 | 50 | 8 | 5 | 62.5 | NS |
| G1 | 17 | 1 | 5.8 | 9 | 3 | 33.3 | < 0.01 |
| G2–3 | 19 | 10 | 50 | 8 | 5 | 62.5 | NS |
| Ta | 23 | 5 | 21 | 10 | 3 | 30 | NS |
| T1 | 12 | 5 | 41 | 7 | 3 | 41 | NS |
| Single | 15 | 5 | 26.6 | 11 | 4 | 36.2 | NS |
| Multiple | 20 | 6 | 30 | 6 | 4 | 66 | NS |

Table 3. Progression rate in relation to DNA content

| | Prophylaxis | | | No prophylaxis | | |
|---|---|---|---|---|---|---|
| | pts | progr. | % | pts | progr. | % |
| Diploid tumor | 19 | – | – | 9 | – | – |
| Aneuploid tumor | 16 | 2 | 12.5 | 8 | 1 | 12.5 |
| Total | 35 | 2 | 5.7 | 17 | 1 | 5.8 |

Table 4. Characteristic of patients with tumor progression

| Pts | Number | Grade | Stage | Ploidy | Prophylaxis | Progression |
|---|---|---|---|---|---|---|
| 1 | single | 2 | 1 | aneupl. | no | 3 months |
| 2 | multiple | 2 | 1 | aneupl. | MYT IFN EPI | 24 months |
| 3 | multiple | 3 | 1 | aneupl. | EPI | 27 months |

rate in aneuploid tumors. Therefore, we can advocate a more conservative approach in the treatment of superficial diploid tumors poorly controlled by TUR (high recurrence rate of widespread localization). In aneuploid tumors, we do not recommend an aggressive approach, because 87.5% of tumors did not progress. If this data is confirmed by a more prolonged follow-up, a search for a more reliable marker or panel of markers of progression is needed.

Comparing other parameters of tumor recurrrence, we found that tumor grading appears to be more reliable as a marker of recurrence than DNA ploidy, even if statistical significance was not reached. When both good grading and diploidy are combined the prognosis for recurrence appears to be most favorable.

Intravesical prophylactic regimens with epirubicin [11], mitomycin C [12] and interferon [13] have been shown to reduce the recurrence rate in 50–70% of the patients. Low-grade, single and primitive tumors appear to benefit most from this therapy [11, 14, 15]. Orihuela et al. [16] showed that BCG intravesical therapy reduces the recurrence rate only in diploid tumors. This observation is confirmed in our study, which shows a good response to intravesical therapy in patients bearing G1 or diploid tumors and an even more favorable one when both these characteristics are associated.

Prophylaxis against progression using intravesical chemotherapy is still controversial. BCG appears to be the only intravesical agent capable of reducing the progression rate of superficial bladder cancer [17, 18]. Sarosdy and Lamm [17] report 4 progressions among 82 patients treated with BCG and followed for 67 months. No definitive data can be drawn for mitomycin C [12]. The absence of progression in the diploid groups after a follow-up of

20 months makes ploidy a reliable marker of tumor progression. If a more extensive follow-up confirms these data, we will be able to modify the follow-up regimen. Our study does not so far provide any data to support a role of intravesical therapy in reducing the progression rate of bladder tumors.

In conclusion, DNA flow cytometry in association with the hystological grade can be a good predictor for bladder tumors that do not progress as well as for response to intravesical therapy in the prophylaxis of tumor recurrence.

## References


1 Barnes RW, Dick AL, Hadley HL, Johnston OL: Survival following transurethral resection of bladder carcinoma. Cancer Res 1977;37:2895–2897.

2 Malmstrom P, Bush C, Norlén BJ: Recurrence, progression and survival in bladder cancer. Scand J Urol Nephrol 1987;21:185–195.

3 Lutzeyer W, Rubben H, Dahm H: Prognostic parameters in superficial bladder cancer. An analysis of 315 cases. J Urol 1982;127:250–252.

4 Gustafson H, Tribukait B, Esposti PL: DNA profile and tumour progression in patients with superficial bladder tumours. Urol Res 1982;10:13–18.

5 Gustafson H, Tribukait B, Esposti PL: DNA pattern, histological grades and multiplicity related to recurrence rate in superficial bladder tumors. Scand J Urol Nephrol 1982;16:135–139.

6 Blomjous CEM, Schipper NW, Baak JPA, van Galen EM, Devoogt HJ, Meyer CJLM: Retrospective study of prognostic importance of DNA flow cytometry of urinary bladder carcinoma. J Clin Pathol 1988;41:21–25.

7 Rubben H, Lutzeyer W, Fischer N, Deutz F, Lagrange W, Giani G, and Members of the Registry for Urinary Tract Tumors, Rheinisch-Westfälische Technische Hochschule, Aachen: Natural history and treatment of low and high risk superficial bladder tumors. J Urol 1988;139:283–285.

8 Soloway MS: Introduction and overview of intravesical therapy for superficial bladder cancer. Urology 1985;36(suppl):18–26.

9 Soloway MS: Rationale for intensive intravesical chemotherapy for superficial bladder cancer. Cancer 1980;44:1050–1058.

10 Devonec M: Une nouvelle hypothèse sur l'histoire naturelle du cancer de la vessie grâce à l'étude du contenu en ADN des tumeurs par la cytométrie en flux. Ann Urol 1987;21:250–256.

11 Blinst Italian Cooperative Group: Intravesical doxorubicin for the prophylaxis of superficial bladder tumors. A multicenter study. Cancer 1984;54:756–761.

12 Huland H, Kloppel G, Feddersen I, Otto U, Brachmann W, Lantzius-Beninga F, Huland E: Comparison of different schedules of cytostatic intravesical instillation in patients with superficial bladder carcinoma: final evaluation of a prospective multicenter study with 419 patients. J Urol 1990;144:68–72.

13 Torti FM, Lum B: Superficial bladder cancer. Risk of recurrence and potential role of interferon therapy. Cancer 1987;59:613–616.

14 Herr HW, Laudone VP, Withmore WF Jr: An overview of intravesical therapy for superficial bladder tumors. J Urol 1987;138:1363–1368.

15 Prout GR Jr, Koontz WW Jr, Coombs LJ, Hawkins IR, Friedell GH, for National Bladder Cancer Collaborative Group A: Long-term fate of 90 patients with superficial bladder cancer randomly assigned to receive or not to receive thiotepa. J Urol 1983;130:677–680.

16 Orihueal E, Varadachay S, Herr HV, Melamed MR, Withmore W Jr: The practical use of tumor markers determination in bladder washing specimens assessing the urothelium of patients with superficial bladder cancer. Cancer 1987;60:1009–1016.

17 Sarosdy M, Lamm DL: Long-term results of intravesical Bacillus Calmette-Guérin therapy for superficial bladder cancer. J Urol 1989;142:719–722.

18 Herr HW, Landom VP, Badalament RA, Friedmann BD, Withmore WF Jr: Bacillus Calmette-Guérin therapy alters progression of superficial bladder cancer. J Urol 1988;139:299A.

Eur Urol 1992;21(suppl 1):31–33

*P. Marandola*[a], *B. Lardennois*[b]
*D. Ploton*[b], *M. Derenzini*[c]
*D. Treré*[c], *B. Campo*[a]
*V. Valentino*[a], *A. Tronci*[a]
*A. Roggia*[a], *P. Broggini*[a]
*D. Vicini*[a], *M. Ruggieri*[a]
*P. Mirando*[a], *C. Iweha*[a]
*A. Speroni*[a]

[a] School of Urology, University of Pavia, Italy;
[b] CHRU, Reims, France, and
[c] University of Bologna, Italy

# A New Marker for Early Detection and Indicator of Progression of Cancer of the Bladder

## Preliminary Results with Ag-NOR Index in 38 Cases of Superficial Bladder Cancer

**Key Words**
Bladder
Prognostic factors
NOR – Nucleolar organizer regions

**Abstract**
The multiform biology of superficial bladder tumors, both morphologically and evolutively, and the lack of reliable predictors of progression have led the authors to study the Ag-NOR proteins as a new marker of these tumors. It is well known that particularly the low-grade superficial tumors frequently relapse on the same histologic and proliferative module. Their potential of progression is probably present at the time of the first manifestation of the disease or it can show itself along the relapsing evolution with classic modifications translating the cellular dedifferentiation.

The NOR index, set up by the authors, has several advantages: firstly, it corresponds to a functional value of normal and neoplastic cells; secondly, it can be used also with paraffin blocks. Another advantage is the semiautomatic lecture, reproducible also in the urinary cytology, mainly of low-grade tumors, reducing the number of false-negatives.

The conclusion of the study of 38 cases of superficial bladder cancer has induced the authors to believe that an increased NOR index is a reliable 'marker' of their progression. Therefore, the authors suggest the use of the NOR activity for the surveillance of the urothelial disease and for a more logical therapeutic strategy.

### Introduction

Superficial bladder tumors occupy a very important place in oncology. Their originality derives from the fact that bladder tumors having similar morphologic appearance have different evolutionary behavior [1]. Some present superficial recurrences while others become infiltrating. The appearance of this event in the natural history of the tumor is a negative prognostic index [2]. The moment of tumor progression is not predictable and cannot be determined during the course of the disease.

The impossibility of evaluating bladder tumor evolution with precision only on the bases of anatomo-morphological and histopathological data has been the stimulus

Prof. Paolo Marandola
School of Urology, University of Pavia
Policlinico S. Matteo
I-27100 Pavia (Italy)


0302–2838/92/0215–0031
$2.75/0

for the search for prognostic indicators to predict tumor behavior [4].

The alterations in nucleolar morphology are constant characteristics already known in neoplastic cells. Neoplastic cells have bigger and irregular nucleoli when compared with those of benign cells. The size and form of the nucleolus are a consequence of the distribution of this gene bearing nucleolar components responsible for the synthesis of ribosomal RNA [3]. These structures are defined as nucleolar organizer regions or NOR. NORs can be visualized by silver staining as they contain argyrophilic proteins called Ag-NOR [5, 6]. These proteins are bound to DNA and play a very important part in the transcription of ribosomal RNA. The intensity of the coloration is an index of cellular proliferation and nucleolar transcription. Nucleolar organizers appear capable of evaluating the initial stage of tumor evolution [3].

**Table 1**

| | Group A | Group B |
|---|---|---|
| Classification | pTa-G1 | |
| Cases | 20 (17 m, 3 f) | 17 (14 m, 3 f) |
| Observation period | 99 months (60–162) | 57 months (18–112) |
| NOR value at pTa-G1 diagnosis | 4.96 | 6.75 |
| Median maximum value | 12.75 | 16.52 |
| NOR value at time of infiltration (pTn-Gn) | – | 9.12 |
| Median maximum value | | 22.00 |

## Materials and Methods

A retrospective study was conducted on 37 patients (31 males and 6 females) with superficial bladder cancer; at onset they all had stage pTa and G1. The following factors were considered: age at the time of diagnosis; the anatomo-clinical characteristics of the initial tumor; the evolution of tumor during 3-monthly cystoscopies prior to resection; the average age of patients before diagnosis was 63.8 years; tumor progression has been variable. Some of the tumors have had recurrences with the same histopathologic characteristics of the primary tumor, others have shown tumor progression by an increase in tumor stage and grade. On the bases of these facts, we have created two patient groups. One group of 20 patients (17 males, 3 females) with primary pTa-G1 in whom recurrence was characterized by infiltration of the basement membrane or bladder muscle as group B.

*Group A:* The average age of patients prior to diagnosis was 57.9 years (youngest at 36 and oldest at 69), and the average follow-up period was 99 months (minimum of 60 months, maximum of 162 months); and 85% of the patients had a recurrence in 5 years.

*Group B:* The average age of the patients before diagnosis is 69.8 years (min. 52, max. 81). The disease-free interval is shorter and recurrences occurred within 2 years in 82% of the patients. The average interval between the initial observation and the appearance of infiltrating disease is 54 months (min. 18, max. 112). The value of Ag-NOR has been obtained from histologic preparations done at the initial time of diagnosis and biopsy samples were obtained from endoscopic resection. Group B patients have been the object of a second reading of Ag-NOR value of the infiltrating process. Group B has two subgroups: B1 before diagnosis (pTa-G1); B2 initial evidence of infiltrating tumor (pTn-Gn). The 54 sliders were read by pathologists (20 of group A and 17 ± 17 of group B) who had no prior knowledge of the clinical history of the patients. The lecture of Ag-NOR values had been done with a semiautomatic method on 100 contiguous neoplastic nuclei; staining was done using Ploton's silver staining technique.

## Results

NOR activity is an index of cellular kinetics, even normal urothelium has its replicative kinetics. It is therefore necessary to define the NOR value of normal urothelium so as to be able to compare it to its neoplastic value, and the mean NOR value for the normal urothelium is 4.5. The mean NOR value for each group is as follows: Group A = 5.89; Group B1 = 7.33, and Group B2 = 9.75.

Comparing the 20 NOR values for group A with the 17 of group B, 37 homologous sections by stage and grade, the difference between group A (5.89) and group B1 (7.33) is statistically significant. It is also statistically significant when group B1 (at initial diagnosis) is compared with group B2 (at initial infiltration) (table 1).

## Discussion

We think that pTa-G1 bladder tumors are best suited to give NOR an index of prognostic value. From a histologic point of view, all papillary proliferations with minimal cellular atypia should be considered carcinomas; pTa tumors are therefore fully fledged carcinomas. G1 tumors have the advantage of being homogeneous compared to G2 and G3, thereby attenuating errors of interpretation. Clinical experience tells us that the majority of well-differentiated tumors shows a benign course while the rest are aggressive. It will be very interesting to know whether such a tumor could contain precocious information about its future significant difference between the tumors of group A and those of group B1; in fact the mean NOR value for group A is 5.89 while that for group B1 is 7.33. On the other hand, the NOR value is higher in group B2 (9.75) than in group B1 (7.33); therefore; the value of NOR increases with tumor infiltration.

Although the NOR value like those of other prognostic indicators of bladder tumors (monoclonal antibodies, Ki 67 and bromodeoxyuridine) should be interpreted as a function of tumor grade and stage, this preliminary study shows that the value of NOR correlates with the histological stage of the primary tumor and with its evolutive potential.

## References


1 Anderstrom C, Johanson S, Nilsson S: The significance of lamina propria invasion of the prognosis of patients with bladder tumors. J Urol 1980;124;23–26.

2 Cairns SP, Suarez V, Newman J, Crocker J: Nucleolar organizer regions in transitional cell tumors of the bladder. Arch Pathol Lab Med 1989;113:1250–1252.

3 Derenzini M, Nardi F: Le regioni nucleolo organizzatrici nucleolari nella diagnosi citologica ed istologica delle neoplasie maligne. Recenti Progr Med 1988;79:463–466.

4 Ooms ECM, Anderson WAD, Alons CL, Boon ME, Veldmujzen RW: Analysis of the performance of the pathologists in the manifestations of grading of bladder tumors. Hum Pathol 1983;14:140–183.

5 Ploton D, Menager M, Janesson P: Improvement in the staining and in the visualization of the Ag-NOR protein (argyrophilic proteins of the nucleolar organizer region) at the optical level. Histochem J 1985;18:5–14.

6 Ploton D, Ménager M, Lechki C: Coloration des organisateurs nuléolaires (NORs) par l'argent. Application à l'étude de la structure du nucléole et intérêt en pathologie. Ann Pathol 1988;8:248–252.

Eur Urol 1992;21(suppl 1):34–36

*Nasser Javadpour*

University of Maryland and Harbor Hospital Center, Baltimore, Md., USA

# Current Status of Tumor Markers in Testicular Cancer

## A Practical Review

**Key Words**
Testis
Marker
Tumor
Cancer
Metastases

**Abstract**
Detection of serum and cellular AFP and hCG has made a significant contribution in understanding and management of testicular cancer. It is essential to remember the following events in utilizing these markers: (1) Histologic diagnosis of seminoma, but AFP is elevated. There is usually an element of choriocarcinoma. (2) Histologic diagnosis of seminoma and highly elevated hCG > 100 ng/ml has usually an element of choriocarcinoma. (3) Histologic diagnosis of choriocarcinoma with an elevated serum AFP. There is usually an element of embryonal carcinoma. (4) Pathologic stage I nonseminomatous testicular cancer with elevated serum markers is either stage II or stage III. (5) In a recent study of 23 patients undergoing resection of residual nonseminomatous testicular cancer after intensive chemotherapy, 21 had either teratoma in primary tumor or bulky metastatic disease. The markers were normalized after chemotherapy and prior to resection. (6) Although normalization of these markers after chemotherapy indicates effective therapeutic response, one should look of residual tumor utilizing radiologic investigations.

Serum and cellular detection of α-fetoprotein (AFP), and human chorionic gonadotropin (hCG) have been established as tumor markers of testicular cancer. This became possible and practical in 1972 when we developed a specific and sensitive radioimmunoassay (RIA) and immunocytochemical technique (ICT) in order to detect a minute amount of these markers in sera and tumor cells of patients with testicular cancer [1, 2]. Although there are a number of markers that are normally produced by embryonic and extraembryonic components of a normal fetus that have been isolated (table 1), AFP and hCG are the most frequent and reliable markers that have become part of the diagnosis, staging, prognosis, and monitoring of this cancer.

### Cell Origin of hCG and AFP

In 1977, utilizing specific and sensitive monoclonal and polyclonal antisera to these markers, the cellular origin of these markers was established in our clinical and laboratory program (table 2). The important fact to remember is that AFP originates from the yolk sac cells, yolk sac tumor cells and yolk sac component of embryonal carcinoma. Also, hCG is produced by syncytiotrophoblastic cells that may be found in seminoma, embryonal carcinoma, teratoma, and yolk sac tumor. hCG is most frequently found in choriocarcinoma, since syncytiotrophoblastic cells are an essential component of this tumor. Ectopic AFP has been reported in benign liver dis-

Dr. N. Javadpour
University of Maryland
22 South Greene Street
Baltimore, MD 21201 (USA)


0302–2838/92/0215–0034
$2.75/0

eases, cancers of the stomach, liver, lung, and pancreas. However, hCG has also been reported in cancers of the lung, liver, pancreas, kidney and bladder. The production of ectopic AFP and hCG does not usually pose a clinical dilemma in the distinction of these cancers from testicular cancer. We have observed elevated serum hCG levels in patients with disseminated bladder and renal cancers. This marker is usually localized in the rapidly growing and frequently undifferentiated cancer cells of these two organs.

### Frequency of AFP and hCG in Testicular Cancer

These markers are mostly found in sera of patients with sufficient tumor bulk and diluted by serum and yet be measured by RIA. The frequency of these markers in testicular cancer is shown in table 2. When measuring the serum levels of these markers, it is important to consider the biologic half-life of hCG (24 h) and AFP (5 days) in the interpretation of these markers.

### Monitoring Therapy

In monitoring the therapy of these tumors, after chemotherapy, surgery and radiotherapy, serial measurements of these markers are essential. It is also equally important to realize that despite returning of these markers to normal level, the patients may still harbor microscopically or radiologically detectable tumors. This particularly happens with chemotherapy, especially in tumors having an element of teratoma. Therefore, in detecting an initial or subsequent residual tumor, it is important to utilize clinical and radiological investigations, in addition to measuring these markers.

It is not unusual to find a discordance between these two markers during chemotherapy. Although normalization of these markers [3, 4] postchemotherapy indicates response of the tumor to chemotherapy, the presence of residual mass, usually detected by radiologic studies, should be resected and serially sectioned [5]. We have several patients who have had elevated serum markers at the conclusion of chemotherapy with residual masses. In 6 patients, our clinical judgement indicated that the resectable masses were the source of these markers and they return to normal levels after resection of the masses. This subset of patients usually benefit from resection of their residual tumors and additional chemotherapy.

### Particular Problems in Seminoma

Although 10% of seminomas have elevated serum hCG, if the serum level is over 100 ng/ml, the tumor may have an element of choriocarcinoma. In such cases, serial sections of the tumor and immunochemical staining for

**Table 1.** Testicular tumor markers

| Specific markers | Nonspecific markers |
|---|---|
| Human chorionic gonadotropin | Lactic dehydrogenase |
| α-Fetoprotein | Carcinoembryonic antigen |
| Placental alkaline phosphatase | Polyamines (putrescine, spermin., spermidine) |
| Placental lactogen | |
| Placental protein Nos 5, 10, 15 | |
| γ-Glutamine transpeptidase | |
| Cell surface antigens | |

**Table 2.** Frequency of elevated hCG and AFP in patients with testicular cancer

| | AFP | | hCG | | AFP and/or hCG | |
|---|---|---|---|---|---|---|
| | pts (n) | % of pts | pts (n) | % of pts | pts (n) | % of pts |
| Seminoma | 2/160 | 0 | 14/160 | 9.0 | 14/160 | 9.0 |
| Teratoma | 6/16 | 37.5 | 4/16 | 25.0 | 7/16 | 43.7 |
| Embryonal carcinoma | 102/145 | 70.3 | 85/145 | 60.0 | 127/145 | 87.5 |
| Embryonal carcinoma with teratoma | 36/56 | 64.2 | 32/56 | 57.0 | 48/56 | 85.7 |
| Choriocarcinoma | 0/5 | 0 | 5/5 | 100.0 | 5/5 | 100.0 |
| Yolk sac tumor | 3/4 | 75.0 | 1/4 | 25.0 | 3/4 | 75.0 |

hCG should solve the problem. Elevated serum AFP in a patient with diagnosis of seminoma almost always indicates the presence of embryonal carcinoma and/or teratoma. Furthermore, other serum markers such as γ-glutamine transpeptidase (GTP) and placental alkaline phosphatase (PAP) may be helpful in diagnosis and management of seminoma.

## Future Perspective

Inclusions of serum LDH, PAP, and GTP may be helpful in a subset of patients, especially those with seminoma and other bulky testicular tumors. The future research should focus on finding additional markers and finding ways to measure these markers with rapid, simple and accurate techniques which are cost-effective.

## References


1 Javadpour N: The role of biologic tumor markers in testicular cancer. Cancer 1980;45:1755.
2 Vaitukaitis JL, Braunstein GD, Ross GT: A radioimmunoassay which specifically measures human chorionic gonadotropin in the presence of human luteinizing hormone. Am J Obstet Gynecol 1972;118:751–758.
3 Javadpour N, Ozolz RF, Anderson T, Gladstein E: A randomized trial of cytoreductive surgery followed by chemotherapy versus chemotherapy alone in bulky stage III testicular cancer with poor prognostic future. Cancer 1982;50:2004–2010.
4 Fossa SD, Aass N, Sigurd O, Hoie J, Stenwif AE, Lien HH, Paus E, Kaalhus O: History of tumor residuals following chemotherapy in patients with advanced nonseminomatous testicular cancer. J Urol 1989;142:1239–1242.
5 Javadpour N, Young JD: Predictors of residual mass requiring surgical resection after chemotherapy of stage III testicular cancer: a prospective study. Urology, in press.

Eur Urol 1992;21(suppl 1):37–38

*T. Zenico*
*M. Zoli*
*M. Fiori*
*F. Fabbri*
*C. Tamburini*
*G. Maltoni*

Division of Urology
(Head: Prof. *G. Maltoni*),
O.C. Morgagni, Forlì, Italy

# Beta-Human Chorionic Gonadotropin and Alpha-Fetoprotein in Central and Peripheral Venous Blood of Patients with Testicular Tumors

**Key Words**
β-Human chorionic gonadotropin
α-Fetoprotein
Venous blood
Testicular tumors

**Abstract**
From January 1989 to June 1991, 18 patients ranging in age from 19 to 41 (mean 34) years with testicular tumor were examined. 14 patients had seminoma (11 typical and 3 spermatocytic) and 4 patients had a mixed form (2 seminoma + embryonal tumor and 2 seminoma + teratocarcinoma). Serum levels of β-human chorionic gonadotropin and α-fetoprotein from peripheral venous blood and from spermatic venous vessel were evaluated in every patient. All patients with seminoma and in a patient with mixed tumor (seminoma + embryonal tumor) the markers were regular. The increase of the markers was found in the peripheral and in spermatic blood of 3 patients (2 seminoma + embryonal carcinoma and 1 seminoma + teratocarcinoma). For these reasons the values of spermatic vessels are an important confirmation of the level of peripheral markers.

## Introduction

β-Human chorionic gonadotropin (β-hCG) and α-fetoprotein (α-FP) are specific markers of malignant neoplasms of the testicle and their importance, from the point of view of diagnosis, staging and monitoring of these tumors, is nowadays a foregone conclusion [1–3]. We thought, however, it would be interesting to look further into the variations in values of these markers by taking central and peripheral venous blood samples [5]. These markers are present in different tumors [2, 4] (table 1). Peripheral applies to the blood taken from the cephalic vein, central to that taken from the spermatic vein during a panorchiectomy.

## Materials and Methods

The study was based on 18 patients under care at our hospital and was carried out during the period January 1989 to June 1991. Of these 18 cases of testicular neoplasia, typical seminomas were diag-

**Table 1**

| | | |
|---|---|---|
| Seminomas | β-hCG 7 | 26% |
| | α-FP 2 | 18% |
| Embryonal carcinoma | β-hCG | 60% |
| | α-FP | 60% |
| Chorion carcinomas | β-hCG | 100% |
| Teratomas | α-FP | 60% |

Dr. T. Zenico
Division of Urology
O.C. Morgagni
I-47100 Forlì (Italy)


0302–2838/92/0215–0037
$2.75/0

**Table 2**

| Patient | Age | Histology | α-FP | | β-hCG | |
|---|---|---|---|---|---|---|
| | | | 0–20 ng | ml% | 0 U | ml% |
| B.G. | 33 | typical seminoma | 0 | 6 | 0 | 0 |
| P.E. | 41 | spermatocytic seminoma | 2 | 4 | – | – |
| U.G. | 40 | typical seminoma | 0 | 2 | – | – |
| C.P. | 30 | typical seminoma | 0 | 10 | – | – |
| S.A. | 25 | typical seminoma | 2 | 12 | – | – |
| S.O. | 37 | typical seminoma | 2 | 2 | – | – |
| S.U. | 19 | spermatocytic seminoma | 3 | 6 | – | – |
| R.E. | 22 | typical seminoma | 0 | 2 | – | – |
| M.M. | 29 | typical seminoma | 2 | 4 | – | – |
| R.M. | 23 | typical seminoma | 0 | 4 | – | – |
| B.M. | 31 | typical seminoma | 2 | 2 | – | – |
| T.L. | 40 | typical seminoma | 3 | 4 | – | – |
| T.V.[1] | 29 | typical seminoma | 2 | 4 | – | – |
| R.R. | 30 | spermatocytic seminoma | 2 | 3 | – | – |
| C.R. | 29 | seminoma + embryonal carcinoma | 3,580 | 17,500 | – | – |
| S.A. | 29 | teratocarcinoma | 182 | 750 | – | 0.5 |
| F.A. | 32 | saminoma+ embryonal carcinoma | 21 | 72 | – | – |
| S.R.[1] | 20 | teratocarcinoma | 100 | 95 | – | – |

[1] Retroperitoneal or inguinal lymphatic metastases.

nosed in 11 patients, spermatocytic seminomas in 3 patients, seminoma + embryonal carcinomas in 2 patients and seminoma + teratocarcinomas in 2 patients. The patients had a median age of 31 (range 19–41) years. All the patients were examined for the presence of β-hCG and α-FP in venous peripheral blood and all underwent panorchiectomies with inguinal incision after an extemporary histological examination. The reflux venous blood was then collected from the funicle in order to quantify the markers present in the central blood. For the patients with seminomas, no markers were found in either of the blood samples. In patients with seminoma + teratocarcinoma as well as those with seminoma + embryonal carcinoma, α-FP was identified in both blood samples, showing a significant increase in the central venous blood (table 2). Only 1 patient (S.R.) showed an increase of markers in peripheral blood (retroperitoneal metastases are present).

## Conclusions

In conclusion, even though relatively few cases have been reported up to the present time, we can still see the high degree of sensitivity of this method, which also gives us the possibility of supplying a diagnostic confirmation and easy comparison of results obtained for the two blood samples. Finally, in using this method, it is also possible to detect the presence of higher marker values in peripheral blood with respect to central blood. In this case, such a finding may indicate the presence of concealed metastases, which then must be further investigated.

## References


1 Di Silverio F: Diagnostica dei tumori testicolari. Aggiorn Androl Chir 1986;1:71–76.
2 Mostofi SK: Testicular tumors: epidemiologic, etiologic and pathologic features. Cancer 1973; 32:1186–1188.
3 Mostofi SK, Price EB Jr: Tumours of the male genital system. Washington, Armed Forces Institute of Pathology, 1973.
4 Javadpour N: Tumor markers in urologic cancer. Urology 1980;16:127–130.
5 Zenico T, Zoli M, Fabbri F, Tamburini C, Maltoni G: Concentrazioni venose spermatiche e periferiche degli ormoni steroidei e gonadotropine in pazienti affetti da varicocele. Atti XII Congresso Nazionale SIRC, 1987, pp 397–402.

Eur Urol 1992;21(suppl 1):39–42

# Characterization of Seven Kidney Tumors by Flow Cytometry: Analysis of Cell Cycle, DNA Content and P-Glycoprotein Expression

*G. Lizard*[a]
*P. Roignot*[b]
*L. Dusserre-Guion*[b]
*F. Morlevat*[b]
*D. Michiels-Marzais*[b]
*N. Ferry*[c]
*J.C. Trémeaux*[d]

[a] Centre Commun de Cytofluorométrie, INSERM U80, Hôpital Edouard-Herriot, Lyon;
[b] Centre de Pathologie et Institut de Recherches Médicales de Bourgogne, Dijon;
[c] Département d'Urologie, Clinique Drevon, Dijon, and
[d] Département d'Urologie, Clinique Ste-Marthe, Dijon, France

**Key Words**
Cell cycle
DNA content
Flow cytometry
Kidney tumors
P-glycoprotein

**Abstract**
Seven kidney tumors obtained from patients aged from 5 to 76 years were analyzed by flow cytometry for cell cycle, DNA content and P-glycoprotein expression involved in multidrug resistance. The DNA index seems to be an important criterion since all the tumors were aneuploid. In a case of clear cell carcinoma, two aneuploid clones were identified. In 5 cases of kidney tumors a high proportion of cells in proliferation (S + (G2 + M)) was observed; it was comprised between 13 and 33%. As for P-glycoprotein it was detected only in few tumor cells (5–15%) respectively in a case of clear cell carcinoma and in a case of Wilms' tumor.

## Introduction

The quantification of DNA content and the study of cell cycle has been widely used in order to predict the evolution of a tumor [1]. Generally, aneuploid tumors are of bad prognosis [2] as well as those with high proportion of cells in proliferation [3]. However, these criteria do not allow to predict the answer of a tumor to chemotherapy and often chemotherapy remains ineffective. Some tumors are intrinsically resistant to chemotherapeutic agents, whereas other tumors can acquire resistance. Sometimes, treatment with one drug may induce the acquisition of resistance to a wide variety of drugs, including structurally and functionally unrelated drugs [4]. This phenomenon is called multidrug resistance (MDR). It is mediated by the overexpression of a 170-kDa membrane protein, the P-glycoprotein (Pgp) which is encoded in human by the two closely related genes, MDR-1 and MDR-2, that encode for highly homologous membrane proteins [5, 6]. Pgp functions as a multidrug transporter that rapidly extrudes many types of chemotherapeutic agents from their target cancer cells before the drugs can exert their cytotoxic effects [7]. Actually, different agents inhibiting the activity of Pgp have been identified and may be of therapeutic interest: anticalcic drugs (verapamil, diltiazem), calmodulin inhibitors, antiarrhythmic drugs (quinidine, amiodarone), tamoxifen and ciclosporin [8]. In normal tissue, Pgp expression has been identified in adrenal, kidney, colon, small intestine and liver [9]. Because of the expression of Pgp in normal kidney, it was of interest to research Pgp in kidney tumors. For these reasons a preliminary study has been realized by flow cytometry on 7 kidney tumor cases. Pgp expression has been revealed with the C219 monoclonal antibody [10] and simultaneously the tumors were characterized with classical methods to precise DNA content and the repartition of the cells in the different phases of the cell cycle.

Dr. G. Lizard
Centre Commun de Cytofluorométrie, INSERM U80
Hôpital Edouard-Herriot, Pav. P
Place d'Arsonval, F–69437 Lyon Cedex (France)


0302–2838/92/0215–0039
$2.75/0

**Table 1.** Histological and flow cytometry characterization of seven kidney tumors without initial therapeutic treatment

| Patient | Age years | Sex | Diagnosis | DNA index | Cell cycle | | | P-glycoprotein % |
|---|---|---|---|---|---|---|---|---|
| | | | | | G0/G1, % | S, % | G2 + M, % | |
| 1 | 76 | F | clear cell carcinoma | 2.08 | ND | ND | ND | 0 |
| 2 | 86 | M | clear cell carcinoma | 1.93 | 80 | 16 | 4 | 5 |
| | | | | 2.19 | ND | ND | ND | ND |
| 3 | 67 | M | clear cell carcinoma | 1.35 | 51 | 29 | 20 | 0 |
| 4 | 5 | F | Wilms' tumor | 1.08 | 80 | 15 | 5 | 15 |
| 5 | 61 | F | angiomyolipoma | 1.09 | 87 | 1 | 12 | ND |
| 6 | 62 | M | clear cell carcinoma | 1.18 | 96 | 1 | 3 | ND |
| 7 | 47 | F | clear cell carcinoma | 2.29 | 70 | 22 | 8 | 0 |

## Material and Methods

*Cell Lines Used*

MCF-7 are human tumor cells of the breast established in culture. Two strains of these cells, one sensible to adriamycin (MCF-7S) and the other one resistant to this drug (MCF-7R), were respectively used as negative and positive control for the expression of Pgp. They were generously provided by Dr. M.F. Poupon (Villejuif, France). The culture medium used for MCF-7S cells was McCoy's with glutamine, insulin and 10% (v/v) fetal calf serum added. MCF-7R were cultured in the same medium supplemented with adriamycin 1.5 μg/ml final concentration. The two cell lines were cultured at 37 °C in a humidified atmosphere containing 5% $CO_2$. To study Pgp expression the cells were used in logarithmic phase and they were subcultured each week by trypsinization with a 0.05% trypsin-0.02% EDTA solution.

*Tumors*

The material studied was obtained from surgery and comprised 7 tumors of the kidney which were initially not treated. For each tumor studied, one part was fixed in 10% neutral formalin and paraffin-embedded for histological typing after staining with hematoxylin-eosin. One other part was frozen in liquid nitrogen to determine DNA content and another one was stored at 4 °C in PBS (pH 7.2) containing sodium azide 0.1% (w/v) final concentration for analysis of Pgp expression.

*Analysis of Cell Cycle and DNA Content*

The collected frozen tumor specimens were minced with a scalpel into mince pieces and treated with hypotonic solutions containing RNase, detergent and propidium iodide [11]. Chicken erythrocytes were used as internal standard [12]. After staining for 30 min, the cell nuclei were filtered through a nylon mesh (40 μm) and run in a FACScan flow cytometer (Becton Dickinson, Mountain View, Calif., USA). The DNA index (DI) was defined as the ratio of the mean channel of the cells of the sample in G0/G1 divided by the calculated mean channel of normal human diploid cells in G0/G1. According to this definition, normal cells are characterized by a DI equal to 1, whereas an aneuploid population is characterized by a DI higher than 1 in case of hyperploidy and a hypoploid population by a DI lower than 1.

*Simultaneous Analysis of Pgp Expression and Cell Cycle*

The tumor specimens were mechanically dissociated and filtered through a nylon mesh (40 μm). The cells were then washed twice in PBS (pH 7.2) without $Ca^{2+}$ and $Mg^{2+}$ and the cell concentration was adjusted at $10^6$ cells/ml. A cell suspension of $10^6$ cells/reaction was treated with the FITC-conjugated C219 antibody diluted 1/20 in PBS (pH 7.2) without $Ca^{2+}$ and $Mg^{2+}$ containing 1% bovine serum albumin (BSA). C219 recognizes a highly conserved cytoplasmic epitope found in all Pgp isoforms and represents a universal probe for Pgp expression [10]. An identical suspension was treated with an antibody, FITC-conjugated $IgG_{2\alpha}$ used at the same dilution, to determine no specific binding. After 30 min incubation in the dark at 4 °C, the cells were washed twice in PBS (pH 7.2) without $Ca^{2+}$ and $Mg^{2+}$ containing 1% BSA. The fluorescently stained cells were then treated with 2.5 μg/ml RNase (Sigma) for 30 min at 37 °C to remove RNA which would affect DNA analysis. The cells were then centrifuged and the cell pellet was treated with 4 μg/ml of propidium iodide (Sigma) for 30 min at 4 °C in the dark before flow cytometry analysis. For flow cytometry analysis the cell concentration in propidium iodide was adjusted at $10^6$ cells/ml and the analyses were run in a FACScan flow cytometer (Becton Dickinson).

*Flow Cytometry Analysis*

Flow cytometry analyses were performed on a FACScan flow cytometer (Becton Dickinson). The excitation source was an argon ion laser emitting a 488-nm beam at 15 mW. The green fluorescence of FITC (λEx max: 494 nm; λEm max: 517 nm) was collected through a 530/30-nm band pass filter, while the red fluorescence of propidium iodide (λEx max: 540 nm; λEm max: 625 nm) was collected through a 585/42-nm band pass filter. 10,000 cells/sample were analyzed. The green fluorescence, related to Pgp expression, was measured on a logarithmic scale and the red fluorescence related to DNA content on a linear scale. The data were analyzed with the software Cellfit (Becton Dickinson) for cell cycle analysis and determination of DNA content, and with the software Lysys (Becton Dickinson) for the expression of Pgp.

## Results

### *Determination of DNA Content and Cell Cycle Analysis*

The DNA content was evaluated according to the value of DI. The higher DIs were observed in clear cell carcinoma (table 1). In the case of clear cell carcinoma corresponding to patients 1, 3, 6 and 7, only one aneuploid population was observed with DI comprised between 1.18 and 2.29. In patient 2, two aneuploid tumoral clones were observed, the first with a DI equal to 1.93 and the second with a DI equal to 2.19 (fig. 1). The lower DIs were found in patients 4 and 5 corresponding to a Wilms' tumor and an angiomyolipoma; they have respectively DI equal to 1.08 and 1.09 (table 1). It is also important to note that in 5 patients (patients 2, 3, 4, 5, 7) high percentages of tumor cells (13–49%) were in proliferation (involved both in S and (G2 + M) phases of the cell cycle) (table 1).

*Flow Cytometry Analysis of Pgp Expression*

Before the study of Pgp expression in kidney tumors, the simultaneous analysis of Pgp expression and cell cycle had been validated. In tumors, this method allows to identify aneuploid clones according to their DNA content and in those conditions to study Pgp expression specifically on them [13]. The method has been validated on two strains of tumor cells of the breast established in culture: MCF-7S sensible to adriamycin and MCF-7R resistant to this drug. Positive cells were identified as follows. Indirect immunofluorescence staining of MCF-7S and MCF-7R cells with the control antibody $IgG_{2\alpha}$-FITC allows to position a vertical cursor which determines the level of no specific immunostaining. All the cells on the left of the cursor were considered negative (fig. 2a, c), whereas all the cells on the right of the cursor were considered positive (fig. 2b, d). In those conditions in strain MCF-7S no resistant cells were identified and in the MCF-7R cells 20% of them strongly

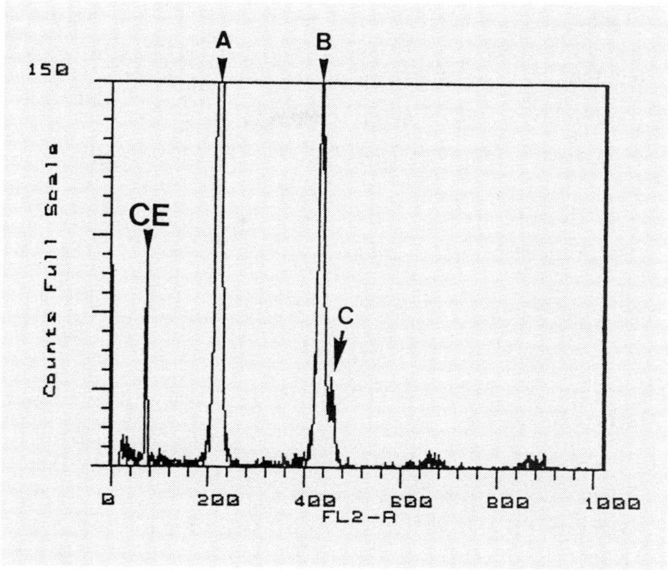


**Fig. 1.** Flow cytometry analysis of cell cycle and determination of DNA content in the case corresponding to patient 2. Chicken erythrocytes (CE) were used as internal standard. Arrow A points towards the G0/G1 peak of normal cells; arrow B points towards the G0/G1 peak position of the first aneuploid clone (DI = 1.93); arrow C points towards the G0/G1 peak position of the second aneuploid clone (DI = 2.19). The cells were stained with propidium iodide and the DNA content was measured on the x-axis on a linear scale from 1,024 channels. The y-axis corresponds to the number of cells per channel (full scale 150 cells).

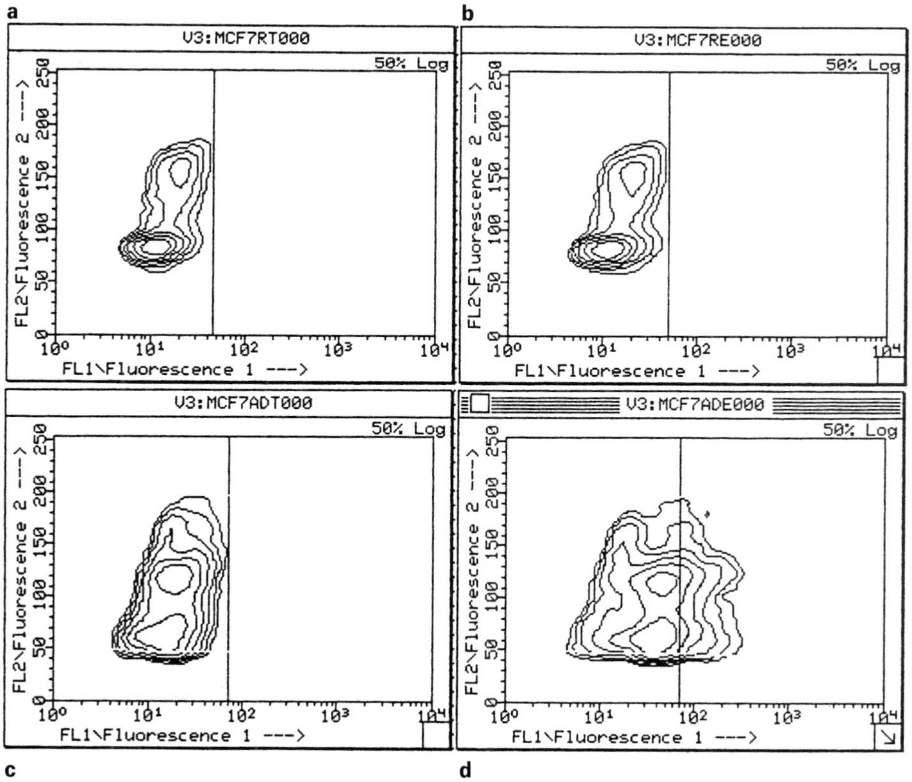


**Fig. 2.** Dual parameter histograms (Pgp expression on x-axis versus DNA content on y-axis) corresponding to the two strains of breast tumor cells MCF-7S and MCF-7R. MCF-7S: **a** $IgG_{2\alpha}$ – FITC versus DNA content (control); **b** C219 – FITC versus DNA content (assay). MCF-7R: **c** $IgG_{2\alpha}$ – FITC versus DNA content (control); **d** C219 – FITC versus DNA content (assay). C219 fluorescence related to Pgp expression is on a log scale and DNA content on a linear scale. The vertical cursor delimits the level between background and Pgp expression. All the cells on the right of the cursor were considered positive. Percent of cells expressing Pgp: 0% in MCF-7S; 20% in MCF-7R.

expressed Pgp whatever their repartition in the different phases of the cell cycle. In our experimental conditions only few cells were found to express Pgp in the kidney tumors studied (table 1). The higher proportion was observed in Wilms' tumor where 15% of tumor cells were positive.

## Discussion

In some types of tumors, specially breast and bladder tumors, abnormal DNA content is considered as being a bad prognosis [1]. In kidney tumors, in agreement with our data, a high frequency of aneuploid tumors were generally observed and aneuploidy seems to be an important prognostic parameter to take into consideration in survival terms [14]. It also appears, among the kidney tumors presently studied, that the percentage of proliferating cells which comprises the cells in the S and G2 + M phases of the cell cycle was particularly high in 5 patients (13–49% of proliferating cells) whereas this proportion in normal tissue is around 5% [15]. It is possible that this increase of cells in proliferation could correspond to tumor aggressivity as previously reported in bladder cancers [16]. Practically, the study of proliferation according to the repartition of the cells in the different phases of the cell cycle by flow cytometry is of interest but remains insufficient to define a chemotherapeutic treatment.

Because of the potential role of Pgp in human cancers [6], its incidence on chemotherapeutic treatment and its expression in normal kidney, Pgp expression was simultaneously analyzed by flow cytometry. In our conditions of analysis, the cells were considered thoroughly positive when their fluorescence was higher than the background. The percentage of positive cells identified in those conditions corresponds to those which strongly expressed Pgp. In the present study all kidney tumors were initially not treated and it appears in those conditions that Pgp-positive cells were detected in low proportions only in two tumors. Such observations can be considered to be in agreement with previous reports since enhancement of Pgp expression in tumors is most often observed after chemotherapeutic treatment [17]. This could explain the lack of Pgp expression in certain kidney tumors where the glycoprotein could be present at a very low level not detectable in our analysis conditions. The proportion of tumors initially containing some cells expressing a high level of Pgp remains to be determined on a larger number of kidney tumors. The eventual expression of Pgp with the DI and the proportion of the cells in proliferation also have to be correlated.

According to these considerations, flow cytometry would constitute a rapid and useful tool in terms of diagnosis and it would also be of interest to apply to patients the most appropriate treatment.

## References


1 Seckinger D, Sugarbaker E, Frankfurt O: DNA content in human cancer. Application in pathology and clinical medicine. Arch Pathol Lab Med 1989;113:619–626.
2 Atkin N, Kay R: Prognostic significance of modal DNA value and other factors in malignant tumors, based on 1,465 cases. Br J Cancer 1979;40:210–215.
3 Kallioniemi O, Punnonen R, Mattila J, Lehtinen M, Koivula T: Prognostic significance of DNA index, multiploidy and S-phase fraction in ovarian cancer. Cancer 1988;61:334–339.
4 Fojo AT, Ueda K, Slamon DU, Poplack DG, Gottesman MM, Pastan I: Expression of a multidrug-resistance gene in human tumors and tissues. Proc Natl Acad Sci USA 1987;84:265–269.
5 Pastan I, Gottesman MM, Ueda K, Lovelace E, Rutherford AV, Willingham MC: A retrovirus carrying an MDR-1 cDNA confers multidrug resistance and polarized expression of P-glycoprotein in MDCK cells. Proc Natl Acad Sci USA 1988;85:4486–4490.
6 Weinstein RS, Kuszak JR, Kluskens LF, Coon JS: P-glycoproteins in pathology: the multidrug resistance gene family in humans. Hum Pathol 1990;21:34–48.
7 Horio M, Gottesman MM, Pastan I: ATP-dependent transport of vinblastine in vesicles from human multidrug-resistant cells. Proc Natl Acad Sci USA 1988;85:3580–3584.
8 Bourhis J, Riou G, Bénard J: Expression de la P-glycoprotéine 170 (GP-170) et résistance à la chimiothérapie des cancers humains. Bull Cancer 1990;77:957–965.
9 Thiebaut F, Tsuruo T, Hamada H, Gottesman MM, Pastan I, Willingham MC: Cellular localization of the multidrug-resistance gene product P-glycoprotein in normal human tissues. Proc Natl Acad Sci USA 1987;84:7735–7738.
10 Georges E, Bradley G, Gariepy J, Ling V: Detection of P-glycoprotein isoforms by gene-specific monoclonal antibodies. Proc Natl Acad Sci USA 1990;87:152–156.
11 Vindelov LL, Christensen IJ, Nissen NI: A detergent-trypsin method of the preparation of nuclei for flow cytometric DNA analysis. Cytometry 1983;3:323–327.
12 Vindelov LL, Christensen IJ, Nissen NI: Standardization of high resolution flow cytometric DNA analysis by the simultaneous use of chicken and tract red blood cells as internal reference standards. Cytometry 1983;3:328–331.
13 Kelsten ML, Berger MS, Maguire HC, Chianese DA, Hellman ME, Weiner DB, Greene MI: Analysis of c-erb-2 protein expression in conjunction with DNA content using multiparameter flow cytometry. Cytometry 1990;11:522–532.
14 Di Silverio F, Gallucci M, Flammia G, Eleutesi P, Moretti T, Cavallo D, De Vita R: Biological and clinical implication of cellular DNA content in renal cell carcinomas. Eur Urol 1991;19(suppl 2):14.
15 Riley RS, Mahin EJ, Perfetto S: DNA analysis; in Clinical Applications of Flow Cytometry. ASCP National Meeting, Las Vegas, Nev 1988, pp 34–57.
16 Devonec M, Darzynkiewicz S, Kostyrka-Claps ML, Collste L, Whitmore N, Melamed M: Flow cytometry of low stage bladder tumors: correlation with cytologic and cytoscopic diagnosis. Cancer 1982;49:109–118.
17 Flier JS, Underhill LH: Multidrug resistance in human cancer. N Engl J Med 1987;316:1388–1393.

Eur Urol 1992;21(supp 1):43–47

*Franco Di Silverio*[a]
*Michele Gallucci*[a]
*Gerardo Paolo Flammia*[a]
*Antonio De Vico*[a]
*Mauro Caponera*[a]
*Patrizia Eleuteri*[b]
*Danilo Forte*[b]
*Delia Cavallo*[b]
*Raffaele De Vita*[b]

[a] Department of Urology, University of Rome 'La Sapienza', and
[b] Environmental Biomedicine Division, ENEA, Casaccia, Rome, Italy

# Biological and Clinical Implication of Cellular DNA Content in Renal Cell Carcinomas

**Key Words**
Flow cytometry
Cellular ploidy
Renal cell carcinoma

**Abstract**
DNA flow cytometric analysis (FCM) was performed on surgical bioptic samples taken from 82 renal cell carcinomas. FCM has evidenced that 35% (29/82) of renal carcinomas resulted diploid, 65% (53/82) aneuploid and of the latter 22% (12/53) multiclonal. Our results do not indicate any relationship among cytometric ploidy, Fuhrman grading, Robson and pTNM staging. A possible interesting increase of aneuploidy frequency was observed between the NMV (66%) subgroup and the no zero NMV (90%) subgroup, while in diploid patients these values were 40% and 10%, respectively. Follow-up data evidence a significant difference in survival pattern of patients between diploid and aneuploid groups. In conclusion, our results show that cytometric ploidy is a potential important prognostic parameter in survival term.

## Introduction

The origin and progression of tumor heterogeneity is defined on the basis of the theory of clonal evolution in tumors proposed by Nowell: tumor progression is the tendency of a neoplasm to worsen in biological and clinical characteristics over time [1]. Flow cytometric analysis (FCM) offers the possibility to describe many aspects of tumoral heterogeneity at the cellular level and to identify new biological parameters for a better characterization of a single neoplasm. The biological origin of renal cell carcinoma (RCC) and behavior of this tumor can be studied with an analytical approach [2, 3]. It is well known that cytometric aneuploidy was observed in many solid tumors and in RCC with spread frequency values; no concordant results, however, were reported on the potentially clinical value of these parameters [4].

The present study was carried out in order to evaluate the biological and clinical significance of cytometric ploidy in association with histopathological follow-up. DNA FCM was performed on surgical bioptic samples taken from 82 RCCs.

## Materials and Methods

*Patients and Histopathological Samples*
Eighty-two consecutive patients underwent simple or radical nephrectomy between January 1983 and July 1991 at the Department of Urology of the University of Rome. Patients' mean age was 57.2 years (± 13.4 SD).

Prof. Franco Di Silverio
Dipartimento di Urologia U. Bracci
Università degli Studi di Roma La Sapienza
Policlinico Umberto I, Viale del Policlinico
I-00161 Roma (Italy)


0302–2838/92/0215–0043
$2.75/0

**Table 1.** Tumor characteristics: Fuhrman grade/ploidy

| Grade (Fuhrman) | n | Ploidy | | | |
|---|---|---|---|---|---|
| | | diploid | | aneuploid | |
| | | n | % | n | % |
| G1 | 15 | 9 | 60 | 6 | 40 |
| G2 | 36 | 10 | 28 | 26 | 72 |
| G3 | 26 | 8 | 30 | 18 | 70 |
| G4 | 5 | 2 | 40 | 3 | 60 |
| Total | 82 | 29 | | 53 | |

**Table 2.** Tumor characteristics: Robson stage/ploidy

| Stage (Robson) | n | Ploidy | | | |
|---|---|---|---|---|---|
| | | diploid | | aneuploid | |
| | | n | % | n | % |
| I | 6 | 2 | 34 | 4 | 66 |
| II | 45 | 20 | 44 | 25 | 56 |
| III | 17 | 3 | 18 | 14 | 82 |
| IV | 14 | 4 | 28 | 10 | 72 |
| Total | 82 | 29 | | 53 | |

**Table 3.** Results: total DNA distribution in 82 patients

| | n | % | Monoclonal | Multiclonal |
|---|---|---|---|---|
| iploid | 29 | 35 | 41 (78%) | 12 (22%) |
| Aneuploid | 53 | 65 | | |

**Table 4.** Tumor characteristics: pTNM stage/ploidy

| pTNM | n | Ploidy | | | |
|---|---|---|---|---|---|
| | | diploid | | aneuploid | |
| | | n | % | n | % |
| | 6 | 2 | 33 | 4 | 67 |
| II | 44 | 18 | 40 | 26 | 60 |
| III | 20 | 6 | 30 | 14 | 70 |
| IV | 12 | 3 | 25 | 9 | 75 |
| Total | 82 | 29 | | 53 | |

*Histopathological Grading*

The morphological grading was performed by our pathologist using the methods proposed by Fuhrman [5] and stage according to Robson et al. [6]. The distribution of grade and stage, both referred to cellular ploidy, is shown in tables 1 and 2.

*Samples*

Renal tissue samples were taken from surgical specimens in areas corresponding to the epicenter and periphery of the lesion and in apparently normal parenchyma. The samples were stored at 4 °C in RPMI 1640 medium (Gibco, New York, N.Y., USA) supplemented with 5% fetal calf serum [7, 8]. Part of these samples were also used for histopathological examination.

First, the samples were washed in physiologic solution (0.9% NaCl). Monocellular suspensions were obtained by mechanical treatment with scissors. The cellular suspensions were fixed with 70% ethanol and stored at 4 °C. Part of the samples were also used for cytologic examination in an attempt to verify their quality for cytometric measurement.

*Flow Cytometric Staining*

The fixed samples were centrifuged at 200 *g* for 10 min and the pellets were resuspended in 0.5% pepsin solution (pH 1.8) for 10 min at room temperature, unter continuous gentle magnetic stirring. The pepsin was then neutralized with 0.1 *M* Tris buffer solution; the samples were centrifuged under the same conditions as before, and the pellets resuspended in the same buffer. The cells were finally stained with a dye solution containing 5 ng/ml ethidium bromide (Serva), 12.5 ng/ml mitramycin (Pfizer Inc., New York, N.Y., USA) and 7.5 m*M* MgCl in 0.1 *M* Tris buffer (pH 7.4) filtered through a 70-nm nylon mesh, and kept at 4 °C for 30–60 min before FCM.

*Flow Cytometry*

The samples were analyzed with a PAS II flow cytometer (Partec, Arlesheim, Switzerland). The signals were collected and accumulated on a 512-channel memory. The histograms were stored on a floppy disk and analyzed by an original software protocol on a PC IBM personal computer. FCM was performed according to the recommendations for DNA cytometry nomenclature [7]. For each case analyzed, the lymphocytes or a normal kidney renal cell sample of the same patient was used as an external and internal standard of cytometrically diploid DNA content. The level of DNA content alteration was ex-

**Table 5.** Tumor characteristics: NMV involvement or not/ploidy

| NMV | Ploidy | |
|---|---|---|
| | diploid, % | aneuploid, % |
| Zero | 44 | 66 |
| No zero | 10 | 90 |

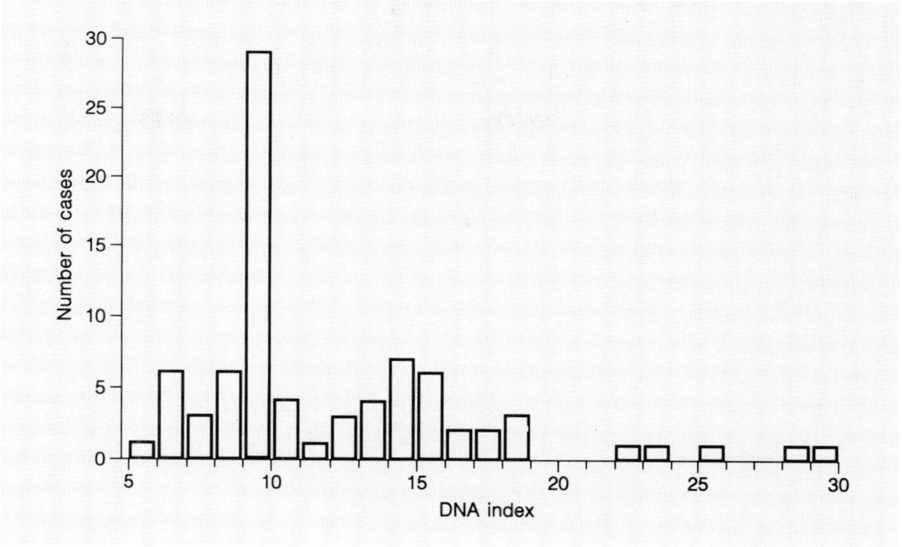


**Fig. 1.** DNA distribution.

pressed in terms of DNA index (DI), evaluated as the ratio of the G1/0 modal values between the aneuploid and diploid subpopulation.

The histogram was defined as diploid when a single population overlapping reference standard was found and when the G2+M cell rate was < 3%. On the other hand, the histogram was defined as aneuploid when one or more populations with peak values other than diploid were found and when the G2+M cell rate was > 3%.

*DNA Histograms and Clinical Data Analysis*

The analysis of DNA histogram data to calculate the cell cycle frequencies (%G1/0, %S1, %G2+M) was performed by a cumulative curve graphic method [12] elaborated on software developed at our laboratory according to the method proposed by Baisch et al. [8]. Statistical analysis of the relationship between cytometric parameters and histopathological and clinical data was performed by the Kaplan-Meier method.

## Results

*DNA Content*

Evaluable histograms were obtained in all cases. In normal samples there was only a diploid cellular DNA distribution, characterized by the occurrence of a G1/0 peak corresponding to 2C DNA content, a G2+M peak corresponding to 4C DNA content, and S-phase cells distributed between the two peaks. A DNA distribution containing only a diploid cell population was found in 29/82 (35%) of the RCCs (table 3). The remaining 53/82 (65%) cases exhibited at least one aneuploid cell subpopulation; of these, 12/53 (22%) were multiclonal and 41/53 (78%) were monoclonal. Thirty-two aneuploid carcinomas (60%) were characterized by the presence of cellular subpopulations with DNA index in the range from 1 to 2 with highest frequency around 1.5. In 16/53 (30%) carcinomas there were hypodiploid subpopulations and in 5/53 (10%) hypertetraploid clones (fig. 1). The average DI value for all aneuploid subpopulations was 1.37 ± 0.54 SD (range 0.5–3.0). In 30 larger carcinomas, epicenter and periphery of the lesion were analyzed to evaluate tumoral heterogeneity in terms of ploidy level. Nineteen of 30 tumors (63.3%) showed the same ploidy in the center and periphery of lesion (7 aneuploid (36.8%) and 12 diploid (63.2%). Heterogeneity was found in 11 of 30 cases (36.7%) and in 8 of them (72.7%), the DNA pattern was diploid. In the remaining 3 aneuploid cases (27.3%), at least one clone characterized by a different DI value was found in one portion of tumor.

*Relationship between Cytometric Ploidy and Pathologic Data*

According to Robson stage, at the time of nephrectomy, 6 cases (7.0%) were stage I; 45 cases (55.0%) stage II; 17 cases (21.0%) stage III (7 IIIa, 6 IIIb and 4 IIIc) and 14 cases (17.0%) stage IV. The relation between Robson stage and ploidy, summarized in table 2, was not statistically significative. Similarly, no significative correlation was found between cellular ploidy and grading; in fact, the occurrence of aneuploid cell subpopulations in G1 group was 40%, in G2 72%, in G3 70% and in G4 60% (table 1). No statistically significative correlation was observed also between ploidy and pTNM stage (table 4). Aneuploidy frequency was 67% in pTNM I, 60% in pTNM II and 70% in pTNM III and 75% in pTNM IV stage. A possible interesting increase in aneuploidy frequency was observed between the NMV (66%) and no zero NMV subgroup (90%) (table 5).

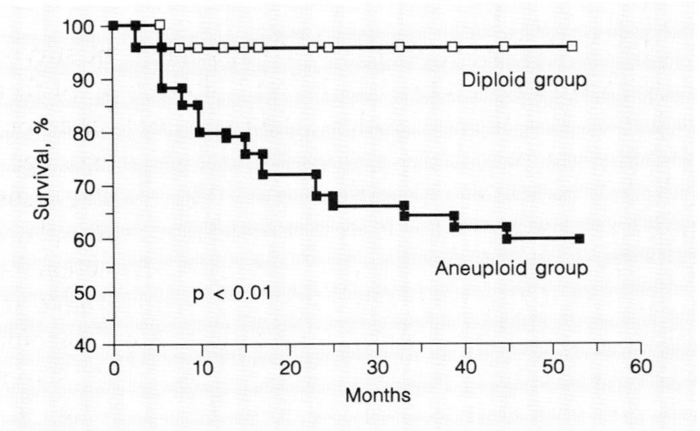


2

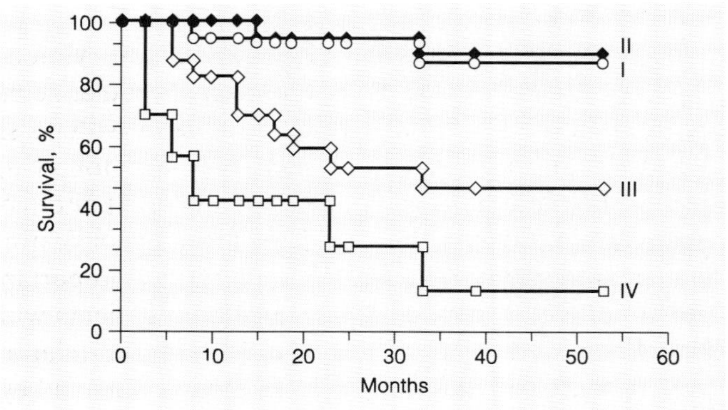


3

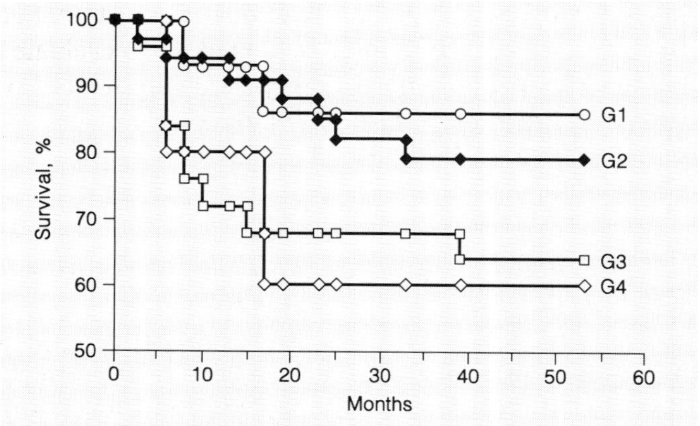


4

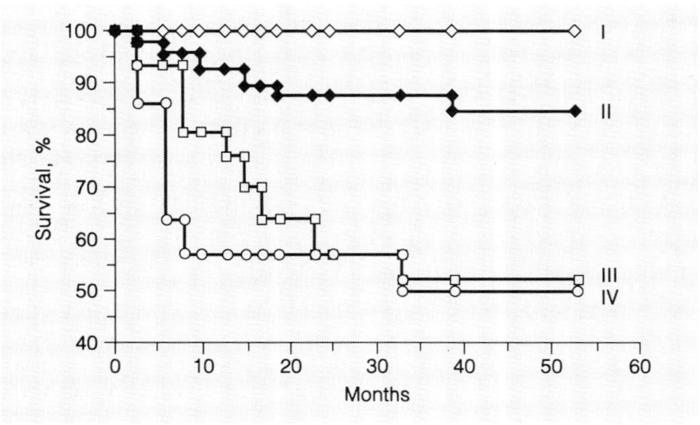


5

*Relationship among Cytometric Ploidy, Pathologic Parameters and Survival*

At present follow-up, all dead patients were characterized by aneuploid tumors with scattered DI value, whereas patients with diploid carcinomas were still alive. The cumulative survival curve of aneuploid cases shows a value of 0.69 (fig. 2). Interesting trends, but not statistically significant, were observed among Robson stage (fig. 3), grading (fig. 4), pTNM stage (fig. 5) and survival. In fact, relevant differences were observed between I–II and III–IV subgroups of renal cell carcinomas.

## Discussion and Conclusions

Several studies have demonstrated the important relationship among grade, clinical stage and survival in RCC patients [3, 9, 10]. Renal vein invasion, genetic and environmental factors are also involved in tumor natural history. Recently, flow cytometry analysis has opened a new chapter in the study of RCC by evaluation of cellular ploidy. Because of RCC's very high cellular heterogeneity [11], we have found it very difficult to set this tumor against a rigid classification. This may be due to the presence of many factors playing a role in tumor aggressiveness and spread. The measurement of DNA ploidy by FCM can furnish further information to the study of cellular heterogeneity. This RCC tumoral characteristic has been confirmed by our results. In fact, we have performed multiple biopsies in 30 larger tumors of the 82 analyzed and in 11 of these (36.7%), FCM analysis evidenced different DI values between tumor center and periphery. The present study showed the occurrence of cytometric aneuploidy in 53 of the 82 (65%) RCC cases analyzed. This frequency is similar to the 63% reported by Ljungberg et al. [12] and is in between the 45% observed by Ljungberg et al. [13] and the 74% reported by Chin et al. [14]. According to numerous other authors, no statistically significative correlation was found among cellular ploidy and histopathological and clinical parameters (Fuhrman grade, Robson stage, pTNM stage) [15]. An interesting relationship was instead observed between cytometric ploidy and invasivity (local and distal); in fact, an increasing aneuploidy frequency was observed in no

**Fig. 2.** Cumulative survival curve/ploidy.
**Fig. 3.** Cumulative survival curve/Robson stage.
**Fig. 4.** Cumulative survival curve/Fuhrman grade.
**Fig. 5.** Cumulative survival curve/pTNM stage.

zero NMV group. The relationship between the survival rate, evaluated by univariate statistic analysis (Kaplan-Meier), and cellular ploidy, Robson stage, pTNM stage and Fuhrman grade, evidenced interesting trends.

*Survival/Ploidy*

A statistically significant correlation among aneuploidy frequency and survival rate was observed. In fact, all dead patients were characterized by aneuploid tumors with scattered DI values, while the patients with diploid DNA content were still alive ($p < 0.05$) at present follow-up.

*Survival/Robson Stage*

An interesting trend, even if not statistically significant, was observed between survival rate in I–II versus III–IV Robson stages patients. In the evaluation of our results, at least two main factors may be considered: (1) the high II stage number (> 50%) of cases probably greatly influences the overall result, and (2) figure 4 shows a sharp spreading apart between stage I–II and stage IV curves. While not statistically significative, it could become positive increasing the number of homogeneous cases.

*Survival/Grade*

Grade I–II neoplasms show a different behavior compared to III–IV grade in terms of clinical outcome. Tumor grade seems to define a clear tendency between the two groups, more evident when follow-up rises above 18 months.

*Survival/pTNM*

Because of the accuracy of pTNM staging, the survival/pTNM ratio turns out to be very interesting. In fact, while no statistically significative difference exists among the various groups, this can be found comparing stage I patients to III–IV stage patients ($p < 0.05$). Such a result can be compared to those present in the literature and it is even more meaningful because lymph node dissection has always been performed. This procedure may have reduced the rate of nodal micrometastases which account for the most part of progression occurring in early stages. A radical and oncologically correct surgery may result in a lower understanding rate and possibly improve the treatment and prognosis.

In conclusion, our results evidenced that the cytometric ploidy can be a useful tool in the study of cellular heterogeneity and clonal evolution of RCC tumors, with possible implications about tumoral behavior. Our follow-up data showed a significant difference in survival pattern of patients between diploid and aneuploid groups indicating that cytometric ploidy represents a potentially important prognostic parameter to identify groups of patients with moderate or low life expectancy. The no correlation among histopathological and clinical parameters and cytometric ploidy suggests a possible role of the latter as an independent parameter in the RCC characterization. Further studies are however requested in order to evaluate a more precise role of cellular DNA ploidy in tumor behavior and eventually in survival of patients.

## References


1 Ljunberg B: DNA content in renal cell carcinoma with reference to tumor heterogeneity. Cancer 1985;56:503.
2 Di Silverio F, La Pera G: Neoplasie del rene; in Mortalità per tumori urologici in Italia: 1971–80. Roma, Acta Medica, 1985.
3 Kaat vander Haute K, Kiss R, de Prez C, et al: Use of computerized cell image analysis to characterize cell nucleus population from normal and neoplastic renal tissues. Eur Urol 1991;19:155–164.
4 De Vita R, et al: Analisi del contenuto di DNA nei tumori solidi umani. Applicazioni cliniche della citometria a flusso. Polo integrato del CNR. Roma, 1989.
5 Fuhrman SA: Prognostic significance of morphologic parameter in renal cell carcinomas. Am J Surg Pathol 1982;665.
6 Robson C, et al: The results of radical nephrectomy for renal cell carcinoma. J Urol 1969;191: 297–303.
7 Hiddeman W, Schumann J, Andreef M, et al: Convention of nomenclature for DNA cytometry. Cytometry 1984;5:445–446.
8 Baisch H, Gohde W, Linden WA, et al: Mathematical analysis of ICP data to determine the fraction of cells in the various phases of the cycle; in Haanen CAM, Hiller HFP, Wessels JMC (eds): 1st Int Symp on Pulse Cytophotometry. Ghent, European Press Medikon, pp 68–76.
9 Rainwater LM, Hosaka Y, Farrow GM, Lieber MM: Well-differentiated clear cell renal carcinoma: Significance of nuclear deoxyribonucleic acid patterns studied by flow cytometry. J Urol 1987;137:15.
10 DeKernion JB: Prognostic significance of DNA content in renal cell carcinoma. Cancer 1989;94:1669.
11 Di Silverio F, De Vita R, Tenaglia R, Forte D, Mauro F, Uccelli R: L'eterogeneità cellulare dei tumori del rene sulla base del contenuto di DNA cellulare determinato mediante citometria a flusso (abstract). Atti XI Congr Naz Oncologia, Bologna, 1985, p 151.
12 Ljungberg B, Steinling R, Roos G: Tumor spread and DNA content in human renal cell carcinoma. Cancer Res 1988;48:3165–3164.
13 Ljungberg B, Stenling R, Roos G: DNA content in renal cell carcinoma with reference to tumor heterogeneity. Cancer 1985;56:503–508.
14 Chin JL, Pontes JE, Frankfurt OS: Flow cytometric deoxyribonucleic acid analysis of primary and metastatic human renal cell carcinoma. J Urol 1985;133:582–585.
15 Nagamori S, Toyota K, Koshiwogi A, Nonomura K, Tahiashianoh M, Kayanagi T: Tumor spread and prognosis in renal cell carcinoma as demonstrated by flow cytometric analysis of deoxyribonucleic acid content. J Urol 1990; 143(suppl):322a, abstr 535.

Eur Urol 1992;21(suppl 1):48–50

Francesco Corrado[a]
Daniele Mannini[a]
Claudio Ferri[a]
Giuseppe Corrado[a]
Franco Bertoni[b]
Patrizia Bacchini[b]
Michael M. Lieber[c]
Jae Mann Song[c]

# The Prognostic Significance of DNA Ploidy Pattern in Transitional Cell Cancer of the Renal Pelvis and Ureter: Continuing Follow-Up

[a] Divisione di Urologia I,
[b] Servizio di Anatomia Patologica,
Ospedale Policlinico S. Orsola-Malpighi,
Bologna, Italia, and
[c] Department of Urology, Mayo Clinic,
Rochester, Minn., USA

**Key Words**
Transitional cell carcinoma
Renal pelvis
Ureter
Flow cytometry
Prognostic factors

**Abstract**
Among 190 patients operated on for transitional cell cancer of the renal pelvis and/or ureter from 1976 to 1990, 95 had their tumor studied by flow cytometry. Of these, the prognostic significance of the DNA ploidy pattern with respect to the standard pathologic features was assessed in a retrospective analysis, where survival information were uptdated to October 1991 and the mean follow-up of patients exceeded 5.5 years (longest follow-up: 15.5 years). Five and ten-year survival probabilities for the whole group were, respectively, 65.5 and 51%. Patients with a diploid tumor had significantly better survival rates than patients with tetraploid/aneuploid cancer ($p < 0.00001$). The impact of the DNA ploidy on survival was confirmed by a multivariate analysis of prognostic factors, where only tumor grade ($p < 0.0001$), tumor stage ($p < 0.0001$), number of neoplastic foci ($p = 0.022$) and nuclear DNA pattern ($p < 0.068$) had a significant influence on survival. In the group of patients with low-stage (pTa-pT1) and low-grade (G1–G2) transitional cell cancer of the upper urinary tract, the DNA analysis was unable to identify any subset of patients at higher risk for disease progression.

## Introduction

As for other malignancies, flow cytometry (FCM) analysis has been suggested to be a useful prognostic tool for transitional cell carcinomas (TCCs) originating from the renal pelvis and ureter. A retrospective study conducted at the Mayo Clinic by Blute et al. [1] on a series of renal pelvis tumors followed for a long time postoperatively, suggested that the DNA analysis of deparaffinized tumor specimens could make it possible to identify patients at risk for disease progression within the group showing moderately differentiated lesions. In a previous study [2] we had attempted a similar analysis on a series of patients treated for TCC of the renal pelvis and/or the ureter: we concluded that, although FCM data were strongly correlated to the outcome of patients, longer follow-up was needed for the group with low-grade and low-stage tumors, to confirm the unfavorable prognostic significance of a tetra/aneuploid pattern. In the present paper we show an update of the same series of patients.

Dr. Daniele Mannini
Divisione di Urologia 1, Ospedale Malpighi
Via P. Palagi, 9,
I-40138 Bologna (Italy)


0302–2838/92/0215–0048
$2.75/0

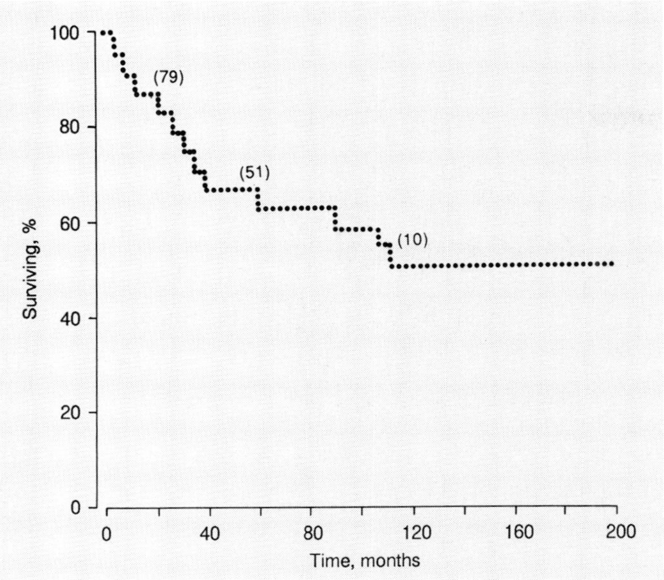


**Fig. 1.** Overall survival of patients (3/95 were lost to follow-up).

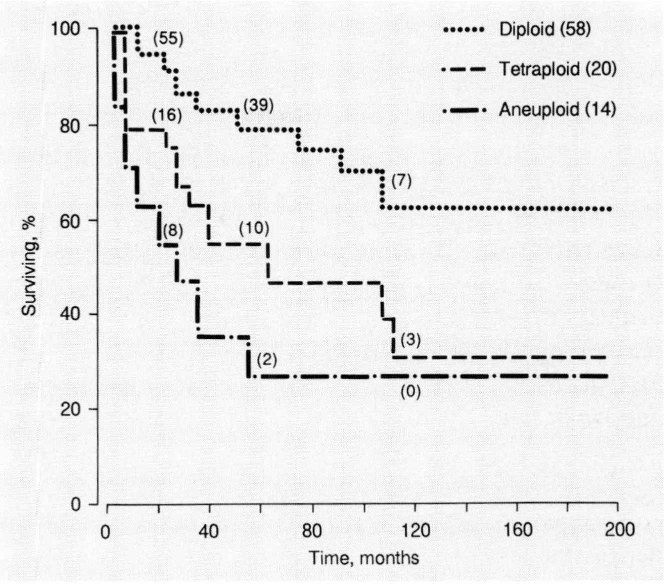


**Fig. 2.** Survival as a function of the DNA ploidy pattern (3/95 patients were lost to follow-up: 2 DNA diploid, 1 DNA tetraploid).

## Material and Methods

From 1976 and 1990, 190 patients were treated surgically for TCC of the upper urinary tract. Tumors were staged following the TNM system [3], and graded according to Broders [4]. In 95 cases it was possible to study the nuclear DNA pattern of the primary tumor: the FCM analysis was conducted at the Mayo Clinic on deparaffinized tumor specimens from archival blocks, following the method described by Hedley et al. [5]. Details about the techniques employed have been described elsewhere [1]. Survival data of the patients were updated to October 1991 and analyzed using the Kaplan and Meier method [6], and the Wilcoxon and Mantel-Cox tests for comparison between two curves [7]. Additionally, a multivariate analysis of possible prognostic factors was carried out using the Cox model [8], assessing the following covariates: age, sex, tumor site (pelvis, ureter), stage, grade, number of neoplastic foci (one or more), DNA ploidy (diploid, tetraploid, aneuploid), association of bladder TCC, kind of surgical treatment employed. For statistical purposes, patients whose cause of death was unknown were considered to have died from cancer and were included in the survival analysis. Further information about materials and methods concerning this series of patients have been published previously [9].

## Results

Three patients were lost to follow-up, 55 were alive and 37 died. Of these, 28 died from TCC and 9 from other causes. The mean follow-up for the whole series of 92 patients was 67.5 months (range 2–196 months). The probability of survival was 65.5% at 5 years, 51% at 10 years (fig. 1).

*Survival as a Function of DNA Ploidy*

As previously reported [10] 60 tumors were classified as diploid, 21 as tetraploid, 14 as aneuploid. Of the 3 patients lost to follow-up, 2 had a diploid and 1 had a tetraploid tumor. The mean follow-up of living patients was, respectively: 86 months for those with diploid tumors (n = 43), 115 months for tetraploids (n = 8), 75.5 for aneuploids (n = 4). Five- and ten-year survival probabilities were, respectively: 79 and 66% for diploids, 55 and 33% for tetraploids. Patients with aneuploid tumors showed a 27% 5-year survival; none of them has yet been followed for 10 years. The comparison between survival curves of diploid tumor patients versus tetraploids and, respectively, aneuploids indicated a highly significant advantage in survival for the diploid group ($p < 0.00001$), while the difference between tetraploids and aneuploids was not significant (fig. 2). When analyzing separately the outcome of 41 patients with low-stage and low-grade disease (pTa-pT1, G1-G2) with respect to the DNA pattern, there was no significant difference between the survival curves of 31 diploids versus 10 tetra/aneuploids, respectively.

*Cox Analysis*

Of the 9 covariates assessed, only 4 were demonstrated to be significantly correlated to the survival of patients, in the following order: tumor grade ($p < 0.0001$), tumor stage ($p < 0.0001$), number of neoplastic foci ($p = 0.022$), DNA ploidy pattern ($p = 0.068$).

## Discussion

The main purposes of our study were : (a) to confirm the usefulness of FCM analysis in the assessment of TCC of the upper urinary tract, which so far had been demonstrated only in one paper from the Mayo Clinic: (b) to verify the hypothesis that FCM can select patients at higher risk of disease progression among those with superficial and moderately differentiated tumors, whose prognosis is otherwise considered to be good.

The fact that in our study the FCM analysis has been also conducted at the Mayo Clinic, with identical method and technology, allowed independent evaluation of clinical and experimental data; in addition, it made possible unbiased comparison of the two studies.

In previous reports [2, 10], we also found that FCM had a powerful impact on prognosis, though its utility as an independent parameter was somewhat limited by the strong correlation it showed with conventional pathologic features, namely the stage and grade of the tumors and their number. As regards low-grade and low-stage tumor patients, we could not observe any significant advantage in survival for those with a diploid pattern, concluding that limited follow-up was one possible pitfall in our analysis. For this reason, follow-up of the whole series was subsequently updated and survival data completely reanalyzed.

At the present time, the mean follow-up of the group of 92 patients with FCM data available exceeds 5.5 years: only 10 of 55 living patients have been followed for less than 5 years, whereby 10 of 55 have been followed for 10 years or more. The survival analysis reported in this paper does not modify significantly our previous results, mainly because no new cancer-related death has occurred in the subset of 10 patients with low-stage, low-grade but tetra/aneuploid tumor.

In conclusion, FCM can be considered as a useful prognostic tool for TCC of the upper urinary tract, though in our series it could not select patients at higher risk for tumor progression among those with low-stage and low-grade disease.

## References

1 Blute ML, Tsushima K, Farrow GM, Therneau TM, Lieber MM: Transitional cell carcinoma of the renal pelvis: nuclear deoxyribonucleic acid ploidy studied by flow cytometry. J Urol 1989;140:944–948.

2 Corrado F, Mannini D, Ferri C, Corrado G, Bertoni F, Bacchini P, Lelli G, Lieber MM, Song JM: Transitional cell cancer of the renal pelvis and ureter: the role of standard pathology and flow cytometry in the prognostic assessment of early diagnosed tumors; in Di Silverio F (ed): Early Diagnosis in Urology. Proceedings of the First Mediterranean Congress of Urology, Rome 1989. Acta Medica, in press.

3 Hermanek P, Sobin LH: TNM classification of malignant tumours, ed 4. Berlin, Springer, 1987, pp 139–141.

4 Broders AC: Epithelioma of the genito-urinary organs. Ann Surg 1922;75:574–604.

5 Hedley DW, Friedlander ML, Taylor IW, Rugg CA,, Musgrove EA: Method for analysis of cellular DNA content of paraffin-embedded pathological material using flow cytometry. J Histochem Cytochem 1983;31:1333–1335.

6 Kaplan EL, Meier P: Nonparametric estimation from incomplete observation. J Am Stat Assoc 1958;53:457–465.

7 Mantel N: Ranking procedures for arbitrarily restricted observations. Biometrics 1967;23: 65–70.

8 Cox DE: Regression models and life tables. J R Stat Soc 1982;34:187.

9 Corrado F, Ferri C, Mannini D, Corrado G, Bertoni F, Bacchini P, Lelli G, Lieber MM, Song JM: Transitional cell carcinoma of the upper urinary tract: evaluation of prognostic factors by histopathology and flow cytometric analysis. J Urol 1991;145:1159–1163.

10 Corrado F, Ferri C, Mannini D, Corrado G, Menniti D, Severini G, Bertoni F, Bacchini P, Lelli G, Lieber MM, Song JM: La citometria di flusso nella valutazione prognostica del carcinoma transizionale dell'alto apparato urinario. Acta Urol Ital 1990;6(suppl 1):227–229.

Eur Urol 1992;21(suppl 1):51–52

*T. Dönmez*
*M. Kale*
*Y. Özyürek*
*H. Atalay*

Department of Urology,
Anadolu University Medical School,
Eskişehir, Turkey

# Erythrocyte Sedimentation Rates in Patients with Renal Cell Carcinoma

**Key Words**
Erythrocyte sedimentation rate
Renal cell carcinoma

**Abstract**
The importance of erythrocyte sedimentation rate (ESR) in patients with renal cell carcinomas (RCCa) is still controversial. ESR levels increased in over half of these patients. In this study, ESR levels of 19 patients with RCCa were investigated (85.368 ± 5.914). In 11 patients in whom carcinomas were only localized in the kidney, the ESR levels were detected as 78.182 ± 8.686. In 8 patients who had metastasis, the ESR levels were found as 95.250 ± 6.427. ESR levels were also estimated in 15 healthy adult persons as control group (18.133 ± 2.180). Mean ESR values were significantly higher in the tumor group than in the control group ($p < 0.01$). There was no statistical difference of the ESR levels between the patients who had local RCCa and advanced RCCa ($p > 0.05$, NS). The removal of the tumoral mass caused the ESR levels to diminish. In conclusion, the ESR levels were not a good criteria in patients with RCCa for evaluating either prognosis or metastasis.

## Introduction

The precise staging and the diagnosis of renal cell carcinoma (RCCa) is made with clinical and radiological investigations and confirmed with pathological evaluations. The main treatment of these tumors is surgery; clinical trials with chemotherapeutic agents or X-ray therapy are disappointing. The prognosis of RCCa is variable: it can regress spontaneously or it can worsen [1]. There is no ideal marker for the diagnosis and follow-up of these tumors. The relationship of serum erythropoietin, lactoferrin, CEA, urine polyamines, serum haptoglobulins, $\alpha_2$-globulins, fibrinogen levels of these renal tumors has been investigated [2–4]. Although there are some studies about cellular androgen and estrogen receptors and cell surface antigens, the clinical importance of these findings has not yet been determined [5]. Erythrocyte sedimentation rate (ESR) is one of these clinical parameters. It has a tendency to increase in cases with renal tumors. The studies to determine the importance of ESR increases in RCCa have led to many comments [6–8].

This study, conducted on patients with renal tumors who had no other health problems, was carried out at the Department of Urology, Anadolu University. The significance of ESR values in renal tumors was investigated.

## Material and Method

In this study, ESR values were detected in the preoperative period in 19 patients with RCCa, the diagnoses of which were confirmed histopathologically. In addition to preoperative investigations, operative evaluations were included in staging of patients with RCCa. Two patient groups, 'localized' or 'advanced', were formed according to their tumors. We also measured ESR levels in 15 healthy subjects as control group. ESR values were measured with the Westergren method [9].

Dr. T. Dönmez
Department of Urology
Anadolu University Medical School
Eskişehir (Turkey)


0302–2838/92/0215–0051
$2.75/0

**Table 1.** ESR values (mm/h) in patients with RCCa and in healthy subjects

| Pat. | Localized tumor group 1 (n = 11) | Advanced tumor group 2 (n = 8) | Healthy subject group 3 (n = 15) |
|---|---|---|---|
| 1 | 18 | 110 | 7 |
| 2 | 115 | 90 | 22 |
| 3 | 65 | 120 | 32 |
| 4 | 80 | 90 | 18 |
| 5 | 96 | 80 | 7 |
| 6 | 75 | 95 | 25 |
| 7 | 86 | 112 | 7 |
| 8 | 95 | 65 | 25 |
| 9 | 80 | – | 22 |
| 10 | 40 | – | 18 |
| 11 | 110 | – | 10 |
| 12 | – | – | 12 |
| 13 | – | – | 15 |
| 14 | – | – | 32 |
| 15 | – | – | 20 |
| | 78.182 ± 8.686 | 95.250 ± 6.427 | 18.133 ± 2.18 |
| | mean 85.368 ± 5.914 | | |
| | ($p > 0.05$, NS) | | ($p < 0.001$) |

## Results

ESR values in patients with renal tumor were found to be 85.368 ± 5.914; in patients with localized tumor (group 1) 78.182 ± 8.686, and in those with advanced tumor (group 2) 95.250 ± 6.427. In healthy subjects (group 3), on the other hand, the ESR value was found to be 18.133 ± 2.80. The difference between patients with renal tumors (groups 1 and 2) and healthy subjects (group 3) is statistically significant ($p < 0.001$), whereas the difference between groups 1 and 2 was not found to be statistically significant.

## Discussion

Hymen and Burns [6] reported in 1950 that ESR levels rose significantly in renal tumors as compared to solitary renal cysts. After this report, many studies were performed on this subject [10]. Besides reports that ESR has a prognostic value, there are others that refute this finding [7, 8, 10–14]. We found the ESR levels to be higher in RCCa patients that in the control group (78.182 ± 8.686 and 18.133 ± 2.189 mm/h, respectively ($p < 0.001$)). Best [15] found in 1987 that ESR levels were high in 43% of cases with renal tumors and Boxer et al. [7] found the same result in 50% of their patients. Ochsner et al. [10] found 50% ESR rise in their series with 103 cases. In a study of 400 cases done at the Mayo Clinic, high levels of ESR were detected in 66% of patients [16]. Woodhouse et al. [4] reported the incidence of ESR rise as 62%. We found in patients with RCCa the ESR rise to be 94% (18/19). It has been observed that some decreases occur after resections of the primary tumor [7]. Fibrinogen, haptoglobulin and $\alpha_2$-globulin levels also increase in patients with renal tumors, some investigators claim that the levels of these parameters correlate with the stage and grade of the tumor, and especially with the extent of metastasis [3]. ESR rises or decreases in protein electrophoresis according to variations in elements other than albumin. Fibrinogen, haptoglobulin, $\alpha_1$-antitrypsin, orosomucoid, ceruloplasmin and serum amyloid a protein are related to α, β, γ fractions of protein electrophoresis and known as acute phase reactants. ESR is a simple and inexpensive measure if it is combined with other parameters in treatment and follow-up of pathologically confirmed renal tumor patients. ESR levels alone do not yield enough information about the course of the disease.

## References


1 Javadpour N: Natural history, diagnosis, and staging of renal cancer; in Javadpour N (ed): Principles and Management of Urologic Cancer, ed 2. Baltimore, Williams & Wilkins, 1983, pp 481–485.
2 Sufrin G, et al: Coagulation factors in renal adenocarcinoma. 1978;119:727–730.
3 Vickers M Jr: Serum haptoglobulins: A preoperative detector of metastatic renal carcinoma. J Urol 1974;112:310.
4 Woodhouse CRJ, Hendry WF, Bloom HJG: Renal carcinoma; in Whitefield HN, Hendry WF (eds): Textbook of Genito-Urinary Surgery. Livingstone, Churchill, 1985, pp 945–961.
5 Bander NH: Comparison of antigen expression of human renal cancer in vivo and in vitro. Cancer 1984;53:1235.
6 Hyman J, Burns E: Significance of the sedimentation rate in urologic disease. J Urol 1950; 64:811.
7 Boxer RJ, Waisman J, Lieber MM, et al: Renal carcinoma: Computer analysis of 96 patients treated by nephrectomy. J Urol 1979;122:598.
8 Hop VCJ, Werf-Messing BHP: Prognostic indexes for renal cell carcinoma. Eur J Cancer 1980;16:833.
9 Raphael SS (ed): Erythrocyte Sedimentation rate; in Lynch's Medical Laboratory Technology, ed 4. Philadelphia, Saunders, 1983, p 694.
10 Ochsner MG, Brannan W, Pond HS, et al: Renal cell carcinoma: Review of 26 years of experience at the Ochsner Clinic. J Urol 1973; 110:643.
11 Bottiger LE: Prognosis in renal carcinoma. Cancer 1970;26:780.
12 Juusela H: Renal adenocarcinoma, clinical features and factors correlating to survival in 173 patients. Ann Chir Gynaecol 1978;67:193.
13 Lieber MM, et al: Renal carcinoma in young adults. Survival and variables affecting prognosis. J Urol 1981;125:164.
14 Skinner DG, Colvin RB, Vermillion CD, et al: Diagnosis and management of renal cell carcinoma. A clinical and pathologic study of 309 cases. Cancer 1971;28:1165.
15 Best BG: Renal carcinoma: A ten-year review, 1971–1980. Br J Urol 1987;60:100–102.
16 Warren MM, Kelalis PP, Utz DC: The changing concept of hypernephroma. J Urol 1970; 104:376.

Eur Urol 1992;21(suppl 1):53–56

*C. Trombetta*
*A. Berretta*
*S. Siracusano*
*M. Gabriele*
*E. Belgrano*

Department of Urology,
University of Sassari, Italy

# Evaluation of Hematochemical Parameters and Renal Echography after ESWL

**Key Words**
Echography
Amylasemia
Creatine phosphokinase
Pseudocholinesterasemia
Serum glutamic-oxaloacetic transaminase
Glutamic-pyruvic transaminase

**Abstract**
Evaluation of hematochemical parameters and renal echography after ESWL treatment with Tripter X1 was done on the first 95 patients treated and for whom we had a longer than 3-month follow-up. Creatinine phosphokinase values showed an increase in 24 patients. 12 patients demonstrated an increase in amylasemia. Echographic checks performed the day after treatment revealed the presence of perirenal lesions in 3 cases. As far as amylasemia is concerned, only 1 patient was treated with aprotinin. One of the patients who developed perirenal hematoma had hypertension; another was following an antiaggregant therapy that was temporarily suspended.

Technological evolution has allowed the creators and constructors to develop lithotripters on the one hand efficient and, at the same time, less complex and less expensive [1]. Our direct experience applies to the Tripter X1, an Israeli-made lithotripter built by Direx Inc.: it is characterized by a system modularity, low initial and running costs and an extreme simplicity of operation [2]. In-depth studies were carried out on the first 95 patients treated and for whom we had a longer than 3-month follow-up. This work covers the characteristics of patients and stones treated, the type of treatment, the results obtained, any complications, and, finally, observations based on *examination of variations in diverse hematochemical parameters.*

We hold that an account of our experience may be useful to Italian urologists insofar as it concerns the first lithotripter of this type used in our country.

## Materials and Methods

The Tripter X1 lithotripter is characterized by the modulatory of its construction. The most important part consists in a shock wave generator (SWAG) on wheels. The patient is placed upon a table designed to facilitate endourological maneuvers. The SWAG is then maneuvered in such a way that its flexible membrane is in contact with the patient's skin surface. The three-dimensional localization of the stone is performed by means of a portable C-arm unit after alignment of the axes to the SWAG. The patient is placed on the X-ray table in such a way as to ensure that the stone be exactly positioned at the focus of shock wave concentration. Once the correct position is obtained, the flexible membrane, which sticks to the patient's skin surface by means of a layer of silicone oil, is inflated. Since the SWAG is quite noisy, both patient and operators are supplied with earphones.

*Patients* (tables 1, 2)
In the period from February to October 1988, we treated 95 patients (41 males and 54 females) whose age varied from 16 to 79. The patients were subjected to 99 treatments insofar as two treatments were necessary in 4 of the cases. The total number of stones treated were 116 (81 patients had a single stone and 14 were carriers of multiple stones).

Dr. Carlo Trombetta
Istituto di Clinica Urologica
Università degli Studi
I-07100 Sassari (Italy)


0302–2838/92/0215–0053
$2.75/0

**Table 1.** Details of tripter X1 treatment performed at the Department of Urology, University of Sassari (Feb.–Oct. 1988)

| | |
|---|---|
| Patients | 95 |
| Stones | 116 |
| Treatments | 99 |
| Kidneys | 95 |

**Table 2.** Age distribution (41 males, 54 females)

| Age group | n |
|---|---|
| 0–20 | 2 |
| 21–30 | 4 |
| 31–40 | 19 |
| 41–50 | 17 |
| 51–60 | 26 |
| 61–70 | 18 |
| 71–80 | 9 |

**Table 3.** kV used during treatments (wide reflector) always 20 kV (min. 190, max. 3,200)

| Shock wave intensity | Shocks per treatment |
|---|---|
| 0–250 | 0 |
| 250–500 | 3 |
| 500–750 | 7 |
| 750–1,000 | 2 |
| 1,000–1,250 | 0 |
| 1,250–1,500 | 9 |
| 1,500–1,750 | 3 |
| 1,750–2,000 | 6 |
| 2,000–2,250 | 29 |
| 2,250–2,500 | 19 |
| 2,500 + | 21 |

**Table 4.** Sizes of the treated stones

| Size, mm | n |
|---|---|
| 5–15 | 51 |
| 15–30 | 26 |
| 30 + | 39 |
| Total | 116 |

*Method* (table 3)

All patients were subjected to shock wave of intensity of 20 kV. The number of shocks per treatment varied from a minimum of 250 to a maximum of 3,200. All procedures were done with the patient under general anesthesia. Auxiliary procedures adopted during treatment were very limited: in 16 cases an ureteral stent was inserted before the procedure; 2 patients had a percutaneous nephrostomy. The length of treatment time varied from 30 to 120 min.

*Characteristics of Treated Stones* (table 4)

51 patients had a less than 15 mm stone; 26 patients had stones of between 15 and 30 mm in size, and in 39 cases stones were over 3 cm in size. 54 patients had a left stone; 72 patients had a kidney stone; in 23 cases the stones were localized at the level of the urether.

## Results

All the patients taken into account were evaluated in the immediate postoperative period and after 3 months by means of echotomography and X-ray tomography. Out of 95 patients, 15 were not present for the follow-up checks and 4 repeated the ESWL treatment during the 3-month follow-up period. Of the remaining 76 patients, 19 (25%) proved to be completely free of fragments when checked by X-ray and echotomography. 21 patients (27.6%) had one or more residual fragments of less than 5 mm in size, often situated in the lower calyx or along the juxtavesical tract of the ureter. These were residual stones susceptible to spontaneous elimination that at the level of the kidney were identified only by means of renal echography. The remaining 36 patients (47.3%) of our initial experience proved to have greater than 5 mm fragments.

If we consider those patients free of stones we can state that: 2 (10.5%) had been treated in presence of a smaller than 15 mm stone; 8 (42.1%) had been treated for stones of a diameter between 15 and 30 mm, and 9 (47.3%) had larger than 30 mm stones.

If we consider stone localization in the 19 patients that resulted 'stone-free' 3 months after the treatment we can see that: in 9 cases the stones were pyelic; in 8 cases they were calyceal (4 localized in the upper calyx, 2 in the middle calyx and 2 in the lower), and in 2 cases the stones were ureteral.

*Complications*

Hematuria was always present. 12 patients had fever (more than 39 °C). No pulmonary or cardiovascular problem (myocardial infarction, cerebrovascular accident) was encountered. In 1 case an asymptomatic pancreatitis was diagnosed on the basis of hematochemical values of amylasemia (see below). Bleeding never required transfu-

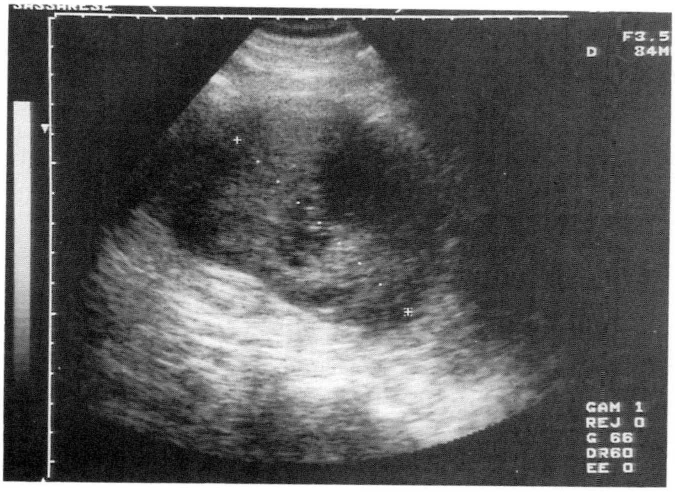


**Fig. 1.** Subcapsular hematoma after ESWL (1,500 shock waves). Echographic check the day after treatment.

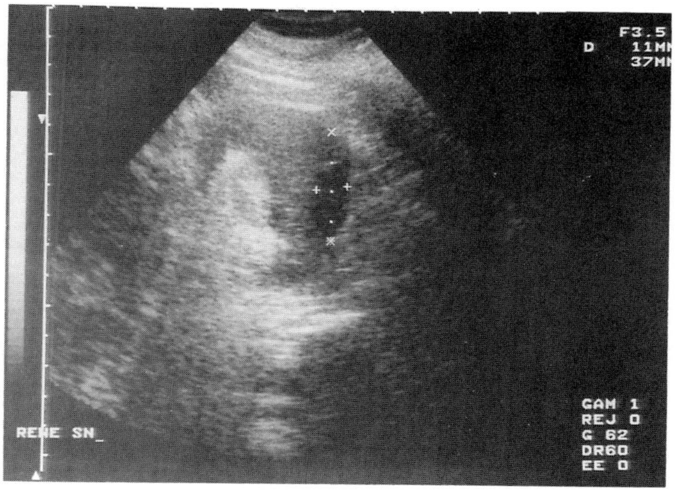


**Fig. 2.** Asymptomatic perirenal lesion occasionally found by means of echography (11 × 37 mm) the day after ESWL treatment with, 3,200 shock waves.

sion. Echographic checks performed the day after treatment revealed the presence of a perirenal hematoma in 3 cases. One of these patients had hypertension (190/110 mm Hg); another was following an antiaggregant therapy (antiplatelets) that was temporarily suspended (fig. 1, 2). 31.5% of patients reported pain after treatment.

*Evaluation of Hematochemical Parameters*

We checked hemochrome, azotemic and creatinemic values, SGOT, SGPT and the hematic levels of amylase, creatine phosphokinase (CPK) and pseudocholinesterase comparing pre- and postoperative levels. As far as amylasemia is concerned, 1 patient who had already had high preoperative levels (242 U/100 ml – normal values: 220 U/100 ml) showed a notable increase arriving at 495 U/100 ml. This patient was treated with aprotinin (Trasylol) 300,000 U intravenously followed by support doses of 50,000 U every 2 h. Another 11 patients demonstrated a slight increase in amylasemia of about 30% starting from low basal levels and remaining within the normal range.

CPK values showed an increase in 24 patients (25%), thereby confirming the muscular tissue involvement and damage during ESWL treatment. 3 patients had an increase in pseudocholinesterase outside the normal range. The majority demonstrated a drop in pseudocholinesterasemia of about 1,000 U. No significant alterations in transaminase values were encountered. Hemochrome, azotemic and creatinemic values did not present any significant variations either.

## Discussion

In evaluating our initial experience with Tripter X1 we sustain that four points must be taken into account: (1) efficacy; (2) analgesic treatment; (3) maneuverability, and (4) costs.

*Efficacy*

Tripter X1 has been able to fragment stones of diverse dimension, form and chemical content into pieces small enough to allow expulsion (in presence of normal excretory pathways). As with other lithotripters, the efficacy of the fragmentation depends upon precision in focusing (and, therefore, upon a good initial localization of the stone), and upon the site of the stone itself and upon its chemical content. The expulsion of fragments varies according to characteristics particular to each patient (efficacy of peristalsis, water load, how long the stone has been in the excretory pathway, etc.). The focusing system of the Tripter X1 is, in our opinion, efficient for all stones of such a dimension to merit treatment. For radiolucent stones we have performed the treatment in the course of urography and/or ureteropyelography. Two patients having cystine stones necessitated a higher number of shock waves, to obtain a good fragmentation and a discrete clearance of stones which were very large.

*Analgesic Treatment*

In our experience we hold that it is better to subject the patient in any case to general anesthesia. The extent of shock wave impact on the patient's skin may be easily noted and evaluated by simply placing a hand between the membrane and the patient's skin: it is of such a degree as to be unbearable over a long period. General anesthesia allows the extension of the treatment for the time necessary to achieve good fragmentation. In addition, the patient remains perfectly still and breathing is regular: thus, all shock waves are aimed solely at the stone, once it is well localized. The constant use of general anesthesia inevitably conditions the choice of ESWL where diverse successive treatments are envisioned for the fragmentation of larger staghorn stones.

*Maneuverability*

This may be considered a weak point of Tripter X1, especially when compared to the computerized systems with which other lithotripters are provided. Focusing times are slightly longer so, as to shorten them and not move the portable C-arm unit, we preferred treating patients all presenting left localized stones during the same sitting. Time is gained, however, during the course of the filling of the membrane which must be stuck to the patient's skin, when compared to lithotripters provided with thanks: in these latter, time is wasted in the changing of the water solution.

*Costs*

The evaluation of the cost-benefit ratio must be considered on two levels: (a) cost-benefit for the patient, and (b) cost-benefit for the institute which acquires the lithotripter. In our opinion, the first point is only apparently of sole clinical interest and, therefore, both must be taken into consideration. Patient evaluation is complex and would necessitate comparative verification among different lithotripters. From our initial experience we sustain that the real handicap lies in the necessity for anesthesia. As far as the relatively minor cost of Tripter X1 is concerned, this allows its acquisition by smaller clinical structures. This would relieve patients of the logistical problems which are quite important in those who have to be treated many kilometers away from the place of residence. These problems include long and uncomfortable trips after treatment and the impossibility of correct follow-ups after ESWL.

## Conclusions

We have concentrated our attention on the follow-ups of patients subjected to ESWL using the Tripter X1. The study of hematochemical parameters has shown an increment of amylasemia in 1 patient who was asymptomatic. The accuracy of echographical follow-up places us in front of data of perhaps less positive a nature but, at the same time, more detailed even as regards renal parenchyma.

## References


1 Servadio C, Livne P, Winkler H: Extracorporeal shock wave lithotripsy using a new, compact and portable unit. J Urol 1988;138:478.

2 Andrianne R, Bonnet P, Bouffioux C, Coppens L, De Leyal J, Similon B: A new generation of renal lithotripters using C-arm fluoroscopy and/or ultrasound stone localization – Tripter X1 (Direx). World Congess on ESWL, Indianapolis 1989, pers. commun.

Eur Urol 1992;21(suppl 1):57–59

L. Veneziano[a], A.R. D'Angelo[b]
L. Burrai[b], G. Perugia[b]
V. Gentile[b], L. Potenza[c]
M.P. Iampieri[c], A. Novelletto[a]
G. Novelli[d], M. Frontali[e]

[a] Dipartimento di Biologia, Università Tor Vergata;
[b] Dipartimento di Urologia, Università La Sapienza;
[c] Dipartimento di Biologia Cellulare e Salute Pubblica, Università di Tor Vergata;
[d] Cattedra di Genetica, Università di Urbino;
[e] Ist. Medicina Sperimentale CNR, Roma, Italia

# DNA Markers in Diagnosis of Adult Dominant Polycystic Kidney Disease

**Key Words**
Autosomal-dominant polycystic kidney disease
Presymptomatic diagnosis
DNA
Genetic heterogeneity

**Abstract**
We report the results of a biological and molecular study carried out on 11 Italian families, with a total of 111 individuals in which adult dominant polycystic kidney disease segregates. A restriction fragment length polymorphism analysis was performed. Two families have shown a genetic heterogeneity even if not phenotypically different from the other ones: they resulted unlinked to 16p markers. A prenatal diagnosis has been performed in a family of the linked type.

## Introduction

In adult dominant polycystic kidney disease (ADPKD) a large number of DNA markers, closely linked to PKD1 on the short arm of chromosome 16, have been detected [1, 2]. This permits an early diagnosis of ADPKD, during the first decades of life, with a specificity of 99%, even in subjects at risk with a negative sonography. However, an estimated 10% of families suffering from ADPKD have shown no evidence of linkage to PKD1. This heterogeneity allows this type of analysis only in large families, with one or more affected members in each generation, in whom it is possible to demonstrate the linkage with DNA markers on chromosome 16.

We report on the finding of two unlinked families in which predictive testing is not yet possible, and on a prenatal diagnosis performed in a linked family.

## Material and Method

Eleven families (111 subjects, 49 patients, 32 at risk 50%, 30 spouses) out of a group of 60 affected by ADPKD collected in Central and Southern Italy were selected to perform a molecular study. Families were selected among outpatients in dialysis centers, urologic and nephrologic departments, and genetic counseling clinics. DNA study was performed in families suitable for linkage analysis selected exclusively on the basis of family size.

Clinical data for each patient of the 11 families were derived from direct clinical and ultrasound examination. DNA was extracted from 20 ml whole blood according to the method described elsewhere [3]. DNA was digested with appropriate enzymes, fractioned in agarose gels transferred to nylon membrane and hybridized with the following probes: 3'HVR.64 [4] and 218EP.6 [5]. Polymorphism 26.6/BstNI-TaqI was performed by enzymatic in vitro amplification of genomic DNA according to Saris et al. [6]. Pairwise and multipoint linkage analyses were performed through a Linkage program [7].

Dr. Anna Rita D'Angelo
Dipartimento di Urologia
Policlinico Umberto
I-00161 Roma (Italy)


0302-2838/92/0215-0057
$2.75/0

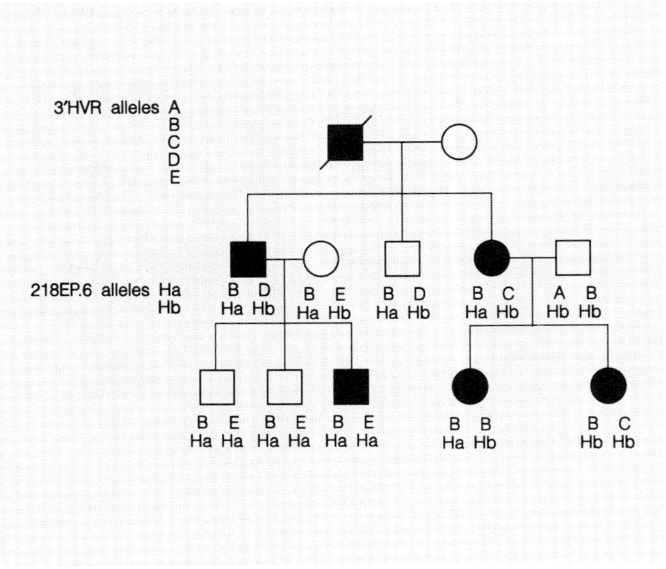


**Fig. 1.** ADPKD family linkage exclusion with 16p markers.

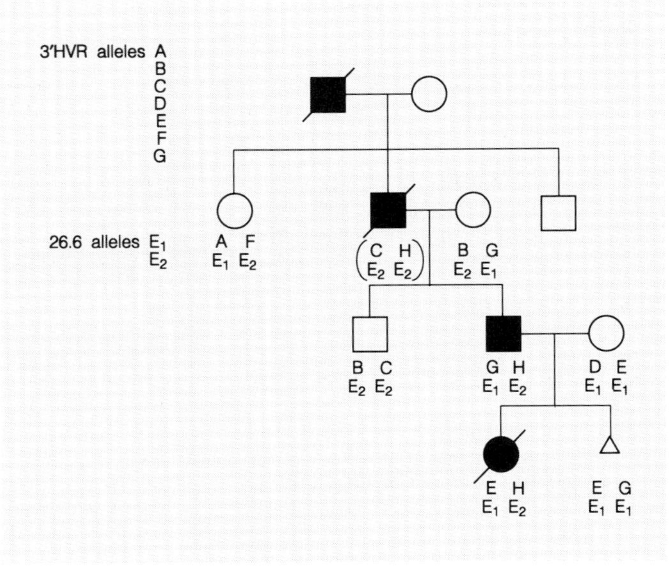


**Fig. 2.** ADPKD family prenatal diagnosis.

*State of the Art*

The advent of recombinant DNA technology permits a novel approach to the study of genetic diseases whose biochemical defect is unknown, as ADPKD. In this approach, termed 'reverse genetic', the mutation producing the disease is first localized by genetic linkage, after that the identification and cloning of the disease gene will allow the understanding of the molecular pathology of this disorder [8, 9].

Another practical advantage of gene mapping is that it allows presymptomatic diagnosis of late onset diseases by an indirect analysis of the disease. Molecular diagnosis of ADPKD is based on the study of the segregation of polymorphic DNA sequences (DNA markers), physically associated to the gene on the chromosome. Such sequences are obtained by cutting DNA with restriction endonucleases. Interindividual differences consist in different sizes of the obtained fragments – restriction fragment length polymorphisms (RFLPs). Since genes closely linked on the same chromosome are inherited together (cosegregate), if there are no recombination events (crossing over) in the chromosome region considered, RFLPs can be used as genetic markers to establish, by segregating analyses, if the disease gene has been transmitted from the affected parent to the son.

At the moment, many PKD1 polymorphic markers are known, which allow ADPKD diagnosis in 95% of the families affected by the disease. Recently, Romeo et al. [10] demonstrated the heterogeneity of ADPKD hypothesizing the presence of a second PKD locus, at the moment still unknown. So we can perform presymptomatic diagnosis of ADPKD only in large families in which we can demonstrate the linkage with the 16p markers. Linkage between the disease and the markers can be demonstrated by calculating lod scores, a likelihood test which compares two hypotheses: one in which we consider the disease linked to the markers, the second in which we consider the disease unlinked.

## Results

In 9 families of our group, linkage between ADPKD and the 16p markers has been demonstrated. Two families showed highly negative lod scores between the disease and these markers: figure 1 shows the pedigree of one of these families. In figure 2 a prenatal diagnosis of ADPKD performed in an informative family is shown. The family was informative for polymorphisms recognized by two flanking markers: 3'HVR and 218EP6. The diagnosis of ADPKD was excluded for the fetus with a probability of 99% and the pregnancy was carried out.

## Conclusion

These results appear to suggest a frequency of heterogenous ADPKD families in Southern and Central Italy of 2/11 (0.18) which is higher than that of 10% so far proposed. A bias in favor of heterogenous families in our sample seems unlikely, since families were selected only on the basis of the number of subjects available for the study. Further investigation on a wider sample of families will be performed in order to confirm the present results.

## References


1 Breuning MH, Snijdewint FGM, Brunner H, Verwest A, Ijdo JW, Saris JJ, Dauwerse JG, Blonden L, Keith T, Callen DF, Hyland VJ, Xiao GH, Scherer G, Higgs DR, Harris P, Bachner L, Reeders ST, Germino G, Pearson PL, Van Ommen GJB: Map of 16 polymorphic loci on the short arm of chromosome 16 close to the polycystic kidney disease gene (PKD1). J Med Genet 1990;27:603–613.

2 Breuning MH, Reeders ST, Brunner H, Saris JJ, Van Ommen GJB: Improved early diagnosis of adult polycystic kidney disease with flanking DNA markers. Lancet 1987;ii:1359–1361.

3 Frontali M, Malaspina P, Rossi C, Jacopini AG, Vivona G, Pergola MS, Palena A, Novelletto A: Epidemiological and linkage studies on Huntington's disease in Italy. Hum Genet 1990;85:165–170.

4 Jarman AP, Nicholls RD, Weatherall DJ, Clegg JB, Higgs DR: Molecular characterization of a hypervariable region downstream of the alpha-globin gene cluster. EMBO J 1986;5:1857–1863.

5 Smidewint FGM, Saris JJ, Dauwerse JG, Breuning MH, Van Ommen GJB: Probe 218EP.6 (D16S246) detects RFLPs close to the locus affecting adult polycystic kidney disease (PKD1) on chromosome 16. Nucleic Acids Res 1990;18:3108.

6 Saris JJ, Breuning MH, Dauwerse JG, Snijdewint FGM, Top B, Fodde R, Van Ommen GJB: Rapid detection of polymorphism near gene for adult polycystic kidney disease. Lancet 1990;335:1102–1103.

7 Lathrop GM, Lalouel JM, Julier C, Ott J: Strategies for multilocus linkage analysis in humans. Proc Natl Acad Sci USA 1984;81:3443–3446.

8 Reeders ST, Breuning MH, Davies KE, Nichols RD, Jarman AP, Higgs DR, Pearson PR, Weatherall DJ: A high polymorphic DNA marker linked to adult polycystic kidney disease on chromosome 16. Nature 1985;317:542.

9 Reeders ST: A 'reverse genetic' approach to autosomal-dominant polycystic kidney disease. Pediatr Nephrol 1987;1:405–410.

10 Romeo G, Costa G, Catizone L, Roncuzzi L, Devoto M, Zucchelli P, Germino GG, Keith T, Weatherall DJ, Reeders ST: A second genetic locus for autosomal-dominant polycystic kidney disease. Lancet 1988;ii:7.

Eur Urol 1992;21(suppl 1):60–65

*Jack A. Schalken*
*Frans M.J. Debruyne*

Department of Urology, Urological Research Laboratory, University Hospital, Nijmegen, The Netherlands

# Identification of New Prostate Cancer Progression Markers by Differential Hybridization Analysis

**Key Words**
Prostate cancer
Progression markers
Differential hybridization analysis
Fibronectin
HMG-I

**Abstract**
In studies on the onset and progression of cancer, molecular biology has proven to be very useful. Reasoning that tumorigenesis can be considered as a multistep process in which a normal cell gradually escapes from its delicately regulated growth pattern, one might describe this process in terms of gene expression. The group of genes that are good candidates for such studies are the proto-oncogenes. Recent progress in oncogene research, however, has made us believe that the group of oncogenes is much greater than the 50 so far characterized, since all growth factor-, growth factor receptor-, signal transducer- and transcription-regulating genes have a potency to become oncogenic. Alternatively, recessive genes, such as tumor suppressor genes, might be equally relevant to the onset and progression of cancer. Therefore, new approaches in molecular studies on the genesis and progression of malignancies are urgently needed. One of these methods is the so-called differential or subtraction hybridization analysis. Particularly, the rationale of differential hybridization and the first applications to prostate cancer research are discussed in this paper.

## Identification of Molecular Characteristics Associated with the Metastatic Ability of Cancer Cells: The Rationale for Differential/Subtraction Hybridization Analysis

The molecular basis of tumor progression can be studied at three levels, i.e. DNA, RNA and protein. The protein expression pattern determines the growth potential, biochemical profile and structural organization of a cell. Aberrant protein expression patterns, leading to cellular transformation and progression, however, can find their origin in genomic alterations. Therefore, studies on the involvement of specific genetic changes, such as chromosomal abnormalities, can serve as a lead to identify genes that are implicated in the onset and progression of cancer [1]. A less complicated technique that is more widely applicable is the so-called allelotyping; DNA probes that map on known chromosomal locations and detect restriction fragment length polymorphisms (RFLPs) can be used to identify consistent deletions of (parts of) chromosomes. Likewise, allelotyping colorectal carcinomas revealed a frequent deletion of the long arm of chromosomes 17 and 18 which led to the identification of p53 and the DCC gene as candidate tumor suppressor genes

Jack A. Schalken, PhD
Department of Urology, Urological Research Laboratory
University Hospital Nijmegen
PO Box 9101, NL-6500 HB Nijmegen (The Netherlands)


0302–2838/92/0215–0060
$2.75/0

[2–4]. The few karyotypes determined from human prostate cancers indicated that the long arm of chromosome 10 (10q23-ter) was deleted in a number of cases [5]. In a recent collaborative study from the departments of urology of the Johns Hopkins Hospital (Baltimore, Md.; Dr. W.B. Isaacs) and the University Hospital Nijmegen, The Netherlands; Dr. J.A. Schalken), the location of two potential tumor suppressor genes implicated in prostate cancer have been identified [6]. We examined 30 prostate cancer specimens for loss of heterozygosity at eleven different chromosomal arms, including chromosomes 3p, 7q, 9q, 10p, 10q, 11p, 13q, 16p, 16q, 17 and 18q. Chromosomes 10p and 16q exhibited the highest frequency of allelic loss. Furthermore, there was an increase in the frequency of allelic loss related to the progressional stage of the disease. Whereas the frequent loss of the chromosomal arm containing the p53 tumor suppressor gene (*17p) which is observed in $>70\%$ of solid cancers is not found in prostate cancer, the loss of 10p and 16q seems to be rather specific for prostate cancer. Chromosomal analyses and allelotyping do not enable us to determine subtle changes in the genome, such as point mutations and/or small deletions. These studies require the use of Southern analyses and/or differential hybridization with oligonucleotides. Such approaches are 'self-limiting', in that respect that they are confined to known genes and/or previously described aberrations. Genes that should be considered relevant are oncogenes, tumor suppressor genes, and genes encoding growth factors, growth factor receptors, transcription factors, extracellular matrix proteins, cell adhesion molecules. The term 'self-limiting', therefore, seems to be an understatement, since taking all this into account, at least 300 known genes should be studied. Studies at the RNA level by Northern blot assays have similar 'constraints; only previously characterized genes can be studied. It should be noted, however, that an overwhelming amount of circumstantial evidence indicates that the above mentioned genes can actually be involved in the onset and progression of cancer. Therefore, the study of these genes and their relation to the etiology and progression of prostate cancer are of major importance.

Just as chromosomal analysis and allelotyping can roughly indicate the genomic location of relevant genes, similar *direct approaches* are necessary to identify proteins that are differentially expressed during the progression of prostate cancer. Unfortunately, no such methods are available yet. Comparison of the protein expression profile by 2D gel electrograms are feasible. Differentially expressed proteins that are thus identified, however, cannot be routinely characterized. Further purification and identification is usually difficult, requiring sophisticated protein technology.

A direct approach to identify genes that are differentially expressed is based on comparison of steady-state mRNA populations, such as differential and subtraction hybridization analyses. These techniques, however, do not enable the identification of genes that are aberrantly expressed (i.e. different size of transcripts). Unless the level of steady-state mRNA has changed, no aberrant expression patterns can be identified. Another constraint of these techniques is that a number of genes can be regulated posttranscriptionally (mRNA stability) or posttranslationally. Such subtle differences cannot be identified using this approach.

The advantages of differential/subtraction hybridization analyses are, firstly, that yet unknown, though relevant genes can be isolated. Moreover, both genes that are up-regulated as well as down-modulated can be identified. Hence, dominant acting genes (e.g. oncogenes, growth factor, and growth factor receptor encoding genes), as well as recessive genetic elements (e.g. tumor suppressor genes) can thus be characterized. Secondly, that the reagents that become available, cDNA clones, can be routinely characterized by DNA sequence analysis and comparison of the resulting DNA sequence with nucleic acid/protein data base. Thirdly, that regardless whether the gene is etiologically related to the disease or (merely) a marker for its progression, the cDNA can be immediately evaluated for its use in diagnosis by RNA in situ hybridization analysis.

Therefore, differential/subtraction hybridization analysis can be a powerful approach to study tumorigenesis and cancer progression. Due to its limitations, however, the technique should be considered complementary to other molecular techniques.

## Applications of Differential/Subtraction Hybridization Analysis to Cancer Metastasis

The above mentioned techniques have been successfully used in the identification of genes induced by growth factors [7–9]. Also genes expressed during the induction of differentiation have thus been identified [10, 11]. Furthermore, comparisons of normal versus malignant tissues using differential hybridization analysis have been successful [12–14].

For metastasis, however, few reports are available on the use of this technique to identify genes that are up-regulated or down-modulated during this process. Inter-

**Table 1.** In vivo biological characteristics of Dunning R-3327 rat prostatic cancer sublines

| Subline | Histology | Growth rate | | |
|---|---|---|---|---|
| | | doubling time days | androgen-responsive | metastatic ability[1] |
| H | well-differentiated | 22±5 | yes | low |
| P | well-differentiated | 10.5±2 | yes | low |
| G | poorly-differentiated | 4.0±0.2 | yes | low |
| CUB | anaplastic | 3.4±0.6 | no | low |
| PAT-1 | anaplastic | 2.8±0.7 | no | low |
| MAT-Lu | anaplastic | 2.7±0.2 | no | high (lungs)[2] |
| AT-1 | anaplastic | 2.5±0.2 | no | low |
| AT-2 | anaplastic | 2.5±0.2 | no | low to moderate (lungs) |
| AT-3 | anaplastic | 1.8±0.2 | no | high (lymph nodes and lungs)[2] |
| PAT-2 | anaplastic | 1.8±0.2 | no | high (lymph nodes and lungs)[2] |
| MAT-LyLu | anaplastic | 1.5±0.1 | no | high (lymph nodes and lungs)[2] |

1 Low metastatic ability, < 5% of s.c. inoculated rats develop distant metastases; moderate ability, > 5%, < 20%; high ability, > 75% develop distant metastases.
2 Organs in the parentheses are the site of the distant metastases for the individual sublines.

estingly, the publications on this topic all report on down-regulation of genes during progression. Our group identified fibronectin as being down-modulated in prostatic cancer cells [15]. Yet another gene, NM23, was down-regulated in melanoma cells with metastatic capacity [16]. WDNM1 is a gene down-regulated in metastatic mammary adenocarcinoma [17]. These results indicate that like in tumorigenesis, suppressor genes might also be involved in metastasis ('metastasis suppressor genes').

### The Dunning R-3327 Rat Prostatic Cancer Model System: The Model System of Choice for Differential/Subtraction Hybridization Analysis?

It should be stressed that the approach of differential hybridization analysis is a powerful one that must be applied to metastasis more frequently in the near future. For such studies, however, a good model system is an essential prerequisite. None of the human in vivo tumor lines available to date exhibit metastatic potential in vivo (after subcutaneous transplantation). For studies on the molecular basis of prostate cancer the Dunning R-3327 rat model system seems to meet the demands for subtraction/differential hybridization analyses.

The parental tumor from which all the rat prostatic tumor sublines were derived, is the original R-3327 tumor described by Dunning [18]. To denote differences in the history of the original R-3327 tumor passaged at several institutes, the tumor line serially passaged at Johns Hopkins Hospital (Baltimore, Md.) was termed R-3327-H. The tumor line passaged at the Papanicolaou Cancer Research Institute (Miami, Fla.) was termed R-3327-P [19]. The P and the H tumor are well-differentiated tumors that grow in response to androgens. The sublines AT-1, AT-2 arose from the Dunning R-3327-H and PAT-1 from the R-3327-P line passaged at Johns Hopkins Hospital [19]. The CUB line was derived from the H line at Dr. Shimazaki's laboratory (Cheba University, Japan) [29]. All these lines arose within one passage and are anaplastic, hormone-independently growing tumors with a low metastatic ability [19], i.e. less than 10% of the animals inoculated with tumor sublines develop distant metastases. MAT-LyLu [21] and MAT-Lu [22] both arose from the AT-1 tumor. PAT-2 and AT-3 arose from the P and H line, respectively. In rats, these last four sublines

**Table 2.** Expression levels measured with pSE-1 as a molecular probe

| Subline | Differentiation | Androgen sensitivity | Metastatic capacity[1] | pSE-1 expression[2] | pBUS expression |
|---|---|---|---|---|---|
| G | poor | sensitive | low | 0 | 0 |
| H | good | dependent | low | 0 | 0 |
| AT-1 | none | independent | low | ++++ | 0 |
| AT-2 | none | independent | low | +++++ | 0 |
| CUB | none | independent | low | ++++ | 0 |
| PAT-1 | none | independent | low | ++++ | 0 |
| MAT-LyLu | none | independent | high | + | ++++ |
| MAT-Lu | none | independent | high | ++ | ++++ |
| AT-3 | none | independent | high | + | +++ |
| PAT-2 | none | independent | high | + | ++++ |

[1] Low, i.e. less than 10% of the animals develop distant metastases; high, i.e. more than 90% of the animals develop distant metastases.
[2] Quantification by densitometric scanning of autoradiographs; 0 = control; level, + = 2 × control level, +++++ = 10 × control level.

grow as anaplastic tumors with a high metastatic ability, i.e. more than 90% of the animals inoculated with these tumor sublines develop distant metastases [19]. The characteristics of the Dunning sublines are summarized in table 1.

The Dunning R-3327 system is a compilation of well-characterized sublines that represent the full spectrum of parameters in which prostate tumor progression can be described (androgen responsiveness, growth rate, histology, metastatic capacity). Hence, we have chosen this system as model for our differential hybridization analyses.

### Identification of Differentially Expressed Genes during the Progression of Prostatic Cancer Cells: A Study on the Dunning R-3327 Sublines

To identify genes whose expression is down-modulated in the process of metastasis, a cDNA library from the anaplastic nonmetastasizing Dunning R-3327 subline, AT-1, was used for a differential hybridization assay, using probes derived from AT-1 and MAT-LyLu mRNAs. MAT-LyLu is a Dunning R-3327 subline that differs from AT-1 in its metastatic capacity, i.e. MAT-LyLu is highly metastatic. The resulting cDNA clones isolated according to the criteria used in a typical differential hybridization experiment were further investigated by using these clones as probes for Northern and dot blots, containing mRNAs of the AT-1 and MAT-LyLu in vitro cell lines. The cDNA clones that detected a differentially expressed mRNA were, subsequently, used as probe on a Northern blot, containing mRNAs of a panel of Dunning tumors that differed widely in their characteristics. The differentially expressed mRNA detected with recombinant clone pSE-1 correlated well with the anaplastic nonmetastasizing phenotype (table 2).

Nucleotide sequence analysis revealed that recombinant clone pSE-1, whose expression was high in all tested anaplastic nonmetastasizing sublines, was identical to fibronectin. To further investigate the down-modulation of this gene, we studied its expression in AT-2.1 and therefrom derived lines that were induced to metastasize by tranfection with the v-Ha-*ras* oncogene [15]. Also during this experimentally induced metastasis, fibronectin mRNA levels were approximately eightfold lowered.

Further improvements in the technique enabled us to increase the sensitivity and the specificity [23]. cDNAs representing 0.01% of the mRNA population can now be detected. Furthermore, the number of clones that appeared to be 'false-positive' in the secondary screening was decreased (10–20%). Thus, the differential screening became more sensitive and efficient.

In a next series of experiments in which we screened for mRNAs that were overexpressed/induced in metastatic prostatic cancer cells, such cDNA clones could be found. A cDNA library of the highly metastatic MAT-LyLu (table 1) was differentially screened with probes representing MAT-LyLu and H (well-differentiated, nonmetastasizing) mRNAs. Upon differential screening of 10,000 recombinant (cDNA insert containing) clones,

> 50 differences were found. In a secondary screening on a panel of three Dunning sublines (i.e. H, AT-2, MAT-LyLu), 20 cDNA clones detected differential expression patterns. Six clones recognized transcripts whose expression level was at least tenfold lower in the H tumor when compared to MAT-LyLu. Those were used as probes to screen ten Dunning R-3327 sublines. It appeared that two clones, pBUS-1 and -19, could specifically discriminate the metastatic tumor lines from the nonmetastatic variants. pBUS-19, however, was not elevated in MAT-Lu, a tumor line that metastasizes exclusively to the lungs. Sequence analysis revealed the identity of these genes.

Thus, two new genes were identified that might be of relevance to the study of prostate cancer etiology and/or progression. Further studies are underway to establish the relevance and usefulness of these genes.

## Discussion and Perspectives

This paper describes the use of differential hybridization analysis to isolate and characterize genes that are upregulated or down-modulated in metastatic prostatic cancer cells. Whether the mRNAs detected with these cDNAs represent genes that are etiologically related to prostate cancer and the progression of the disease, or (merely) a marker for progression/metastasis, remains to be established.

The obvious next steps are the cloning of the genes and transfection on recipient cells. This could be under its own promotor or heterologous (inducible) promotor. Evaluation of transfectants can give a clue to the causal relation between the overexpression/down-modulation of the gene and the metastatic phenotype.

If the thus identified genes are only a marker of progression of the disease, clearly they could still be of great value. Diagnosis of prostate cancer is still hampered by the lack of such markers that predict the relative aggressiveness of an individual tumor. The need for such 'progression markers' is further indicated by the fact that most likely more localized cancers (i.e. stage A-2, B-1,2) will be clinically diagnosed in the near future, due to the improvement of diagnostic tools (e.g. transrectal ultrasound) and the screening of population groups at risk (males > 50 years old). Taking all this into account, the primary clinical application of cDNAs identified by differential hybridization analyses might very well be to determine the individual aggressiveness of a tumor on the basis of its expression pattern.

The mRNA abundancy threshold of the differential hybridization assay, > 0.01% (i.e. only cDNAs detecting mRNAs that are expressed at more than 0.01% of the total mRNA population will be identified), indicates that the reagents can be used immediately in diagnosis: either in RNA in situ hybridization or by Northern blot analysis of mRNA extracted from pathologically defined tissue.

Clearly, to use this technique for the identification of molecular progression markers in other urological cancers, a well-characterized model system will be essential. For bladder cancer, for instance, no well-described model system that represents the steps implicated in the progression from papillary tumors to invasive disease is yet available. Similar constraints are noticable for renal cell carcinoma. It will therefore be critically important to define systems which are a potential starting point for differential/subtraction hybridization studies, since we think that the results obtained to date confirm the applicability of this technique to cancer research. Many new aspects of tumorigenesis and cancer progression are expected to be defined at the gene expression level using this approach. Moreover, important new diagnostic agents are likely to become available.

## References


1 Yunis Y: Chromosomal basis of neoplasia. Science 1983;221:227–236.

2 Hinds Ph, Finly C, Levine A: Mutation is required to activate the p53 gene for cooperation with the *ras* oncogene and transformation. J Virol 1989;63:739–746.

3 Baker SJ, Fearon ER, Nigro JM, Hamilton SR, Preisinger AC, Jessup JM, Van Tuinen P, Ledbetter DH, Barker DF, Nakamura Y, White R, Vogelstein B: Chromosome 17 deletions and p53 gene mutations in colorectal carcinomas. Science 1989;244:217–221.

4 Fearon E, Cho K, Nigro J, Kern SE, Simons JW, Rubbert JM, Hamilton SR, Preisinger AC, Thomas G, Kinzler K, Vogelstein B: Identification of a chromosome 18q gene that is altered in colorectal cancers. Science 1990;247:49–55.

5 Atkin NB, Baker MC: Chromosome study of five cancers of the prostate. Hum Genet 1985; 70:359–364.

6 Carter BS, Ewing CM, Ward WS, Treiger BF, Aalders TW, Schalken JA, Epstein JI, Isaacs WB: Allelic loss of chromosomes 16q and 10q in human prostate cancer. Proc Natl Acad Sci USA 1990;87:8751–8755.

7 Almendral JM, Sommer D, MacDonald-Bravo H, Burckhardt J, Perera J, Bravo R: Complexity of the early genetic response to growth factors in mouse fibroblasts. Mol Cell Biol 1988;8:2140–2148.

8 Lau LF, Nathans D: Identification of a set of genes expressed during the $G_0/G_1$ transition of cultured mouse cells. EMBO J 1985;4:3145–3151.

9 Lau LF, Nathans D: Expression of a set of growth-related immediate early genes in Balb/c 3T3 cells: coordinate regulation with c-*fos* or c-*myc*. Proc Natl Acad Sci USA 1987;84:1182–1186.
10 Kartasova T, Cornelissen BJC, Belt P, Van de Putte P: Effects of UV, 4-NQO and TPA on gene expression in cultured human epidermal keratinocytes. Nucleic Acid Res 1987;15: 5945–5962.
11 Smits HL, Floyd EE, Jetten AM: Molecular cloning of gene sequences regulated during squamous differentiation of tracheal epithelial cells and controlled by retinoic acid. Mol Cell Biol 1987;7:4017–4023.
12 Augenlicht LH, Kobrin D: Cloning and screening of sequences expressed in a mouse colon tumor. Cancer Res 1982;42:1088–1093.
13 Yamamoto M, Maehara Y, Takahashi K, Endo H: Cloning of sequences expressed specifically in tumors of rat. Proc Natl Acad Sci USA 1983; 80:7524–7527.
14 Matrisian LM, Bowden GT, Kriegg P, Furstenberger G, Briand JP, Leroy P, Breatnach R: The mRNA coding for the secreted protease transin is expressed more abundantly in malignant than benign tumors. Proc Natl Acad Sci USA 1986;83:9413–9417.
15 Schalken JA, Ebeling SB, Isaacs JT, Treiger B, Bussemakers MJG, De Jong MEM, Van de Ven WJM: Down-modulation of fibronectin mRNA in metastasizing rat prostatic cancer cells revealed by differential hybridization analysis. Cancer Res 1988;48:2042–2046.
16 Steeg PS, Bevilacqua GB, Kopper L, Thorgeirsson UP, Talmadge JE, Liotta L, Sobel ME: Evidence for a novel gene associated with low tumor metastatic potential. J Natl Cancer Inst 1988;80:200–204.
17 Dear TN, Ramshaw IA, Kefford RF: Differential expression of a novel gene, WDNM1, in nonmetastatic rat mammary adenocarcinoma cells. Cancer Res 1988;48:5203–5209.
18 Dunning WF: Prostate cancer in the rat. Monogr Natl Cancer Inst 1963;12:351–369.
19 Isaacs JT: Development and characterization of available animal model system for the study of prostatic cancer; in Coffey DS, Bruchovsky M, Gardner WH, Resnick MI, Kerr JP (eds): Current Concepts and Approaches to the Study of Prostatic Cancer. New York, Liss, 1987, pp 513–576.
20 Minagawe H, Miyauchi T, Wakisaka M, Susi H, Matsuzaki O, Shimazaki J: Properties of two sublines derived from rat prostatic adenocarcinoma (Dunning R-3327 tumor). GANN 1983;74:524–533.
21 Isaacs JT, Yu G, Coffey DS: The characterization of a newly identified, highly metastatic variant of the Dunning R-3327 rat prostatic adenocarcinoma system: The MAT-LyLu tumor. Invest Urol 1981;19:20–23.
22 Lazan D, Heston WD, Kadman D, Fair W: Inhibition of the R-3327 MAT-Lu prostatic tumor by diethylstilbestrol and 1,2-bis(3,5-dioxopiperazin-1-yl)propane. Cancer Res 1982; 42:1390–1394.
23 Bussemakers MJG, Debruijne FMJ, Van de Ven WJM, Schalken JA: Identification of HMG-I(Y) as potential progression marker for prostate cancer by differential hybridization analysis. Cancer Res 1991;51:606–611.

Eur Urol 1992;21(suppl 1):66–70

*Anna de Matteis*

Department of Human Biopathology,
Section of Pathological Anatomy,
University 'La Sapienza', Rome, Italy

# Tissue Markers in the Diagnosis and Prognosis of Prostatic Carcinoma

**Key Words**
Prostate
Carcinoma
Tissue markers
Diagnosis
Prognosis

**Abstract**
Prostatic acid phosphatase (PAP), prostate-specific antigen (PSA), and β-microseminoprotein are organ-specific markers. Also Leu-7 may be regarded as an organ-specific marker. The main utilization of PAP and PSA immunostaining is to establish the prostatic origin of a carcinoma. Changes of PAP and PSA immunoreactivity may be correlated with histologic grade of prostatic carcinoma. Keratin expression assessment is useful to identify prostatic basal cells or epithelial secretory cells. Neuroendocrine marker reactivity in prostatic carcinoma seems to be related with increasing histologic grade and tumor progression.

Usually the histological diagnosis of prostatic carcinoma does not offer any difficulty. However, artifactual histologic figures in small tissue sample or microscopic areas of well-differentiated adenocarcinoma may be mis taken for atrophy, adenomatous atypical hyperplasia (AAH) [1], basal cell hyperplasia [2] or other prostatic lesions.

The prognosis correlates well with histologic grade, size and stage of prostatic carcinoma but more precisely predictive parameters are continuously explored for improving management of individual patients. Unfortunately, a single immunohistologic marker for diagnosis and prognosis of prostatic carcinoma is not available at present. According to some authors, useful information may be inferred from the evaluation of multiple antigens, comparing carcinoma and benign prostate [3].

This brief exposition is focused only on the most commonly used prostatic tissue markers.

## Organ-Specific Markers

Besides the well-known prostatic acid phosphatase (PAP) and prostate-specific antigen (PSA), other organ-specific markers, such as β-microseminoprotein (β-MSP or β-inhibin), can be used [4–6]. Moreover, Leu-7, a differentiation antigen of the natural killer cells, also recoghizes prostatic epithelial cells and may help to identify the prostatic origin of a metastatic carcinoma, even though with some limitations [7–9].

PAP and PSA are the more used prostatic tissue markers being commercially available, highly specific and sensitive and giving optimal results with routinely formalin-fixed and paraffin-embedded specimens. PAP corresponds to the isoenzymes of the acid phosphatase exclusively produced by the prostate. Acid phosphatase enzymatic activity has been evaluated in serum and detected in tissues of prostatic origin [10–12] for many years prior to the advent of specific immunologic methods [13, 14]. The cognizance of PSA, a neutral protease biochemically and immunologically distinct from PAP, is more recent [15]. However, PSA quickly achieved larger acceptance

Dr. A. de Matteis
Dipartimento di Biopatologia Umana
Sezione di Anatomia Patologica, Policlinico Umberto I
Viale Regina Elena, 324, I-00161 Roma (Italy)


0302–2838/92/0215–0066
$2.75/0

than PAP because of its remarkable specificity. Quantitative evaluation of serum levels of PSA is pervasively employed for clinical diagnosis and monitoring of prostatic carcinoma, on the basis of the strong correlation between its high serum concentration and occurrence of prostatic carcinoma. Therefore, serum PSA can be regarded as a circulating tumor marker. However, tissue detection of PAP and PSA have a different meaning. These two enzymes are produced by the secretory epithelial cells of normal, hyperplastic and malignant prostate, so corresponding to organ-specific markers.

Immunostainings reveal positive fine granules of PAP or PSA within the cytoplasm of the secretory epithelial cells with no significant difference between normal and hyperplastic prostate (fig. 1). The staining is prevalent in the supranuclear area on the luminal aspect of the cytoplasm where apical blebs may be observed. Secretion in the acinar lumen is also stained. Some difference in the staining intensity among the cells may be observed, with occasionally unstained cells. The prostatic basal cells, underlying the secretory cells in benign acini, do not synthesize PAP or PSA and are completely negative with immunostaining for these antigens (fig. 2) [16]. Also, epithelial cells of seminal vesicle and prostatic urethra are unreactive with antibodies anti-PSA and anti-PAP.

The usual prostatic adenocarcinoma retains the ability to synthesize PAP and PSA at least as long as it preserves sufficient differentiation (fig. 3, 4). The epithelial cells in the differentiated prostatic adenocarcinoma show a cytoplasmic staining as do the benign cells but the range of immunoreactivity from cell to cell and from sample to sample may be broader than in benign prostate.

Ultrastructural investigations demonstrate PAP to be a lysosomal enzyme [17] and PSA localized in cytoplasmic vacuoles, vesicles, secretory granules and endoplasmic reticulum of the secretory epithelial cells in benign and malignant prostate [17, 18]. In the poorly differentiated carcinomas, with impairment of the cytoplasmic organelles, PSA may be associated with membrane structures. Interestingly, in carcinoma and, to a lesser extent, in benign hyperplasia, PSA is also detected in stromal macrophages and in circulating neutrophils, suggesting the possibility of different ways of transport in normal and in pathological conditions [18].

A number of investigations concern the correlations of tissue PAP or PSA with histologic grading in prostatic carcinoma [5, 16, 19–24]. The results are not uniform. However, the prevalent data indicate a great heterogeneity of the immunoreactivity, a reduced staining intensity and a decreased number of positive cells in moderately and poorly differentiated carcinoma. Some poorly differentiated prostatic carcinomas show loss of antigenic activity for PAP or PSA or both. The concomitant use of PAP and PSA immunostaining in adjacent tissue sections improves the sensibility of the method, which achieves about 100%. In our experience, at least a focal positive PSA or PAP immunostaining is almost always detected in poorly differentiated carcinomas, when adequate sampling is available. Nevertheless, a very small number of undifferentiated prostatic carcinomas certainly lack PSA and PAP immunoreactivity.

In the daily practice, the main aim of PSA and PAP immunohistochemistry is to establish the tumor histogenesis. The positive PAP and PSA immunostaining in the carcinoma with endometrioid features (so-called endometrial carcinoma) has provided evidence for a prostatic origin of this previously presumed müllerian tumor [25–29]. Moreover, in this tumor the positive PSA or PAP staining allows a differential diagnosis with transitional cell carcinoma originating from urethra or prostatic ducts.

PSA and PAP detection is fundamental to distinguish between primary or secondary carcinoma of the prostate and to verify the prostatic origin of an unknown metastatic tumor [21, 30–32]. However, negative staining reactions do not immediately exclude the prostatic origin of a carcinoma, especially with undifferentiated carcinomas which may be unreactive in spite of their prostatic origin. Moreover, when the immunoreactivity is focal, a small specimen may be negative, not being representative of the whole tumor. Also, previous therapy has to be considered as possible cause of loss of immunoreactivity [33, 34].

The sensitivity of PAP of PSA may be affected by the use of monoclonal or polyclonal antibodies, the source and purity of the antisera and some technical factors [22].

The specificity of PAP is somewhat lower than that of PSA. Positive immunoreaction for PAP has been reported in islet cell tumor of the pancreas [35], breast carcinoma [36], intestinal carcinoid [37, 38], renal cell carcinoma [36], adenocarcinoma of the urinary bladder [39]. PSA is considered highly specific. However, positive tissue staining has been observed in normal apocrine sweat glands, sweat gland apocrine carcinoma and apocrine breast carcinomas, when polyclonal antibodies are used, whereas the reaction is negative with monoclonal antibodies [40].

Discrepancies between PSA serum levels and degree of tissue immunoreactivity may be sometimes observed. Morphology cannot completely explain this and biochemical modifications and changes in mechanisms of the cell product transport are probably involved.

**Fig. 1.** PSA immunostaining of hyperplastic prostate. Positive granules are more abundant at the apical aspect of the cytoplasm.

**Fig. 2.** PSA immunostaining of basal cell hyperplasia. The basal cells are negative; only a few luminal cells are stained.

1

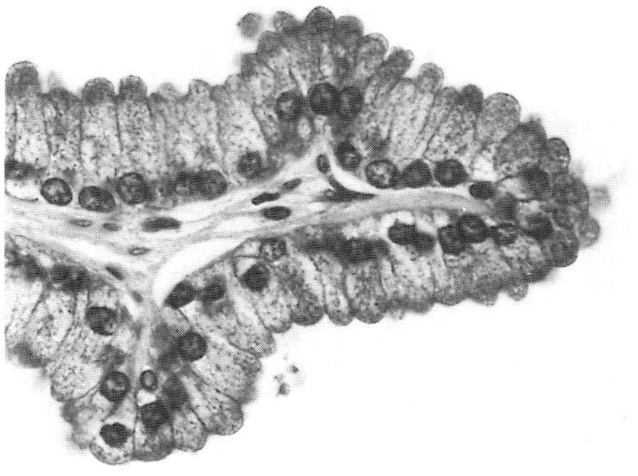

2

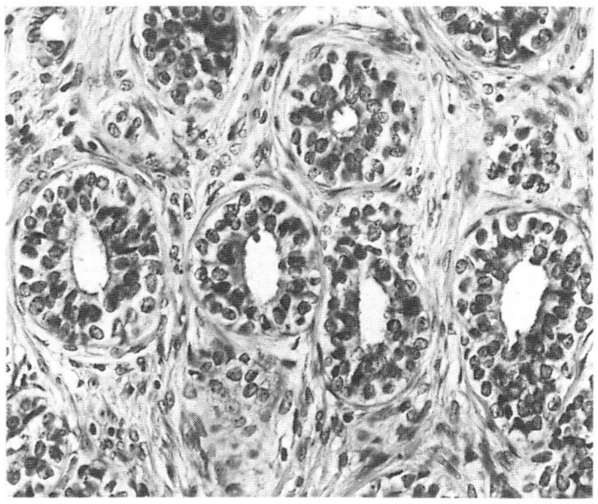

**Fig. 3.** PAP immunostaining of a moderately differentiated adenocarcinoma. Staining heterogeneity of the cells is evident.

**Fig. 4.** Positive PSA immunostaining of poorly differentiated adenocarcinoma; cells surrounding lumina are more deeply stained than other cells.

3

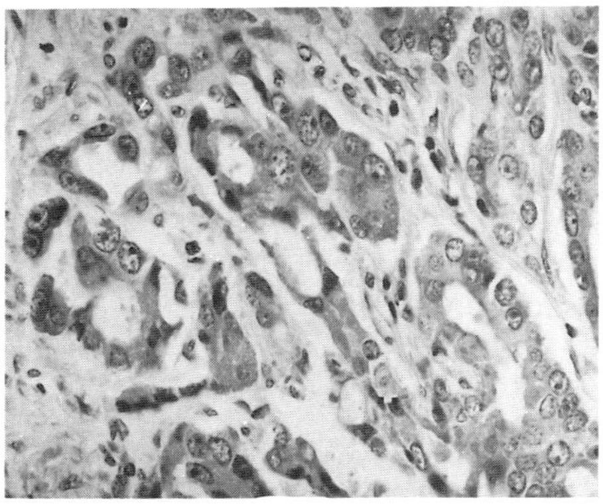

4

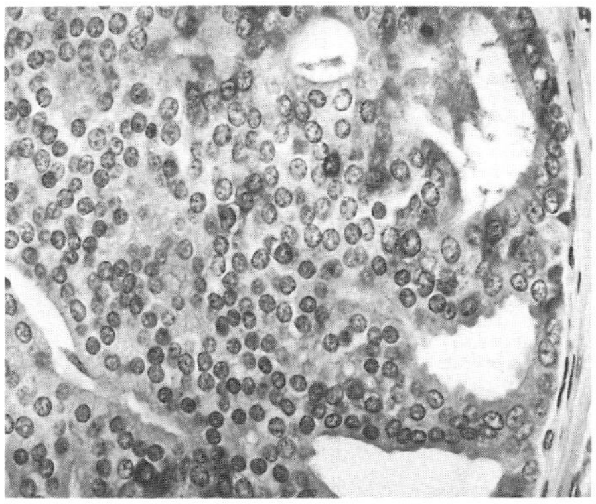

**Fig. 5.** Stratum corneum keratin immunostaining of hyperplastic prostate. Only basal cells are stained.

**Fig. 6.** Chromogranin immunostaining of a poorly differentiated prostatic adenocarcinoma with neuroendocrine differentiation.

5

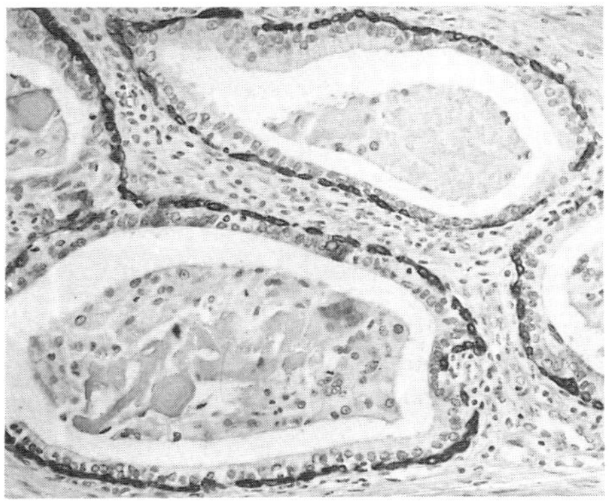

6

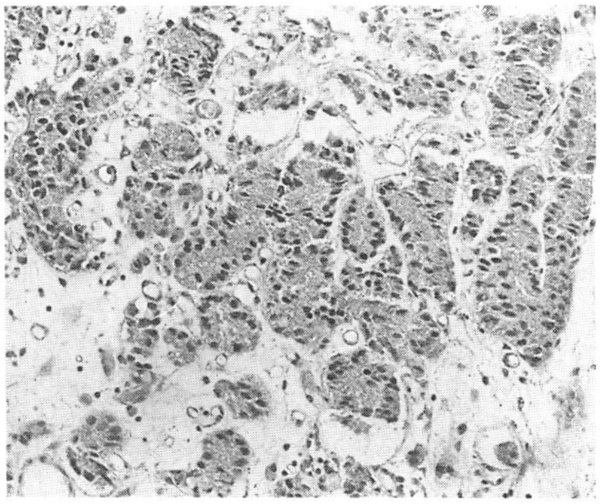

## Intermediate Filament Proteins

Keratins (or cytokeratins) are the intermediate filament's proteins of the epithelial cells, distinguished in 19 subclasses and 2 subfamilies according to the molecular weight and isoelectric pH [41]. Each type of epithelium and corresponding tumors express a peculiar set of keratins, so assuming immunohistochemical identity. In the prostate, keratins from human stratum corneum are detected exclusively in the basal cells whereas keratins typical of the simple epithelia, between which the number 8 and 18, are present in the secretory cells only [42–44]. A continuous basal cell layer stained with appropriate keratin antibodies characterizes benign acini (fig. 5), being completely or partially lost in carcinoma or prostatic intraepithelial neoplasia (PIN) [45]. Basal cell hyperplasia and the rare and disputed prostatic adenoid cystic carcinoma share the same antigenic profile with basal cells, thus making proper identification easier [46].

Adenocarcinoma of the prostate expresses the same keratins as do the normal secretory cells but changes in staining properties have been reported, with similarity between invasive carcinoma and PIN [47]. Vimentin, the intermediate filaments of tissues of mesenchymal origin, may be coexpressed by the epithelial cells in benign prostate and adenocarcinoma [44].

The comparative analysis of the reports concerning specific keratins expressed by the single epithelial types and tumors may offer some difficulty due to use of immunochemical or histochemical procedures and different antibodies which can be broadly reactive or very specific. Moreover, immunostaining of keratins is significantly influenced by the choice of the fixative. Indeed, formalin fixation and paraffin embedding do not guarantee preservation of the immunoreactivity. With specimens so processed, the use of proteolytic enzymes considerably enhances the tissue immunoreactivity.

### Neuroendocrine Markers

It is well known that endocrine/paracrine cells are present in the normal prostate and in benign prostatic hyperplasia. The use of neuroendocrine markers, such as neuron-specific enolase (NSE), chromogranins, synaptophysin, has allowed to achieve retrospective evaluation of archival paraffin blocks of prostatic carcinomas [48–50]. Primary prostatic carcinoid tumors or small cell carcinomas, pure or mixed with areas of conventional adenocarcinoma, have been observed [51–53]. Moreover, occurrence of neuroendocrine differentiation in conventional prostatic carcinoma (fig. 6) has been also reported, prevalently in poorly differentiated carcinomas. Positive PSA and PAP immunostainings have been detected in areas of carcinoid [54] whereas small cell carcinoma of the prostata lacks PSA and PAP immunoreactivity [52].

The number of neuroendocrine cells seems to be proportional to increasing grade of anaplasia during progression of the prostatic carcinoma [55]. Moreover, the emergence of prostatic small cell carcinoma may occur in a previously diagnosed conventional adenocarcinoma regardless of its initial grade [51]. On this basis, the finding of neuroendocrine cells in prostatic carcinoma could have prognostic implications and the value of a progression marker. The increased number of neuroendocrine cells during tumor progression may be almost partially explained by the selective action of the traditional therapies, with overgrowth of the unresponsive neuroendocrine component. An autocrine function of the endocrine cells with resultant excessive proliferation is also regarded as highly probable [56].

### Other Prostatic Tissue Markers

Carcinoembryonic antigen (CEA) is not effective in the diagnosis of prostatic carcinoma being prevalently negative in this lesion. Pepsinogen II (PG II) and tissue plasminogen activator (t-PA) have been detected in the epithelial cells exclusively pertaining to prostatic central zone. However, the epithelial cells of the peripheral zone may also express these antigens when duct-acinar dysplasia (PIN) or carcinoma are present [57]. PG II and t-PA could work as tumor markers for malignant lesions of the peripheral zone of the prostate, namely the most part of them.

Immunoreactivity of cell surface blood group antigens with monoclonal antibodies is not significantly different in nodular hyperplasia and carcinoma [58] whereas with specific red cell adherence techniques a complete loss of reactivity has constantly been observed in prostatic carcinoma [59].

### References


1 Bostwick DG, Srigley JR: Premalignant lesions; in Bostwick DG (ed): Pathology of the Prostate. Contemp Issues Surg Pathol. New York, Churchill Livingstone, 1990, vol 15, pp 37–59.
2 Cleary KR, Choi HY, Ayala AG: Basal cell hyperplasia of the prostate. Am J Clin Pathol 1983;80:850–854.
3 Rubenstein M, Shaw MW, Ray V, Dubin A, McKiel CF, Guinan P: Application of immunohistologic staining to develop a malignant index to aid in distinguishing benign from malignant prostatic tissue. Prostate 1989;14:383–388.
4 Lilja H, Abrahamsson P-A: Three predominant proteins secreted by the human prostate gland. Prostate 1988;12:29–38.
5 Abrahamsson P-A, Lilja H, Falkmer S, Wallström LB: Immunohistochemical distribution of the three predominant secretory proteins in the parenchyma of hyperplastic and neoplastic prostate glands. Prostate 1988;12:39–46.
6 Aumüller G, Seitz J, Lilja H, Abrahamsson P-A, von der Kammer H, Scheit K-H: Species- and organ-specificity of secretory proteins derived from human prostate and seminal vesicles. Prostate 1990;17:31–40.
7 Rusthoven JJ, Robinson JB, Kolin A, Pinkerton PH: The natural-killer-cell-associated HNK-1 (Leu-7) antibody reacts with hypertrophic and malignant prostatic epithelium. Cancer 1985;56:289–293.
8 Wahab ZA, Wright GL: Monoclonal antibody (anti-Leu-7) direct against natural killer cells reacts with normal, benign and malignant prostate tissue. Int J Cancer 1985;36:677–683.
9 May EE, Perentes E: Anti-Leu-7 immunoreactivity with human tumours: its value in the diagnosis of prostatic adenocarcinoma. Histopathology 1987;11:295–304.
10 Gomori G: Distribution of acid phosphatase in tissues under normal and under pathological conditions. Arch Pathol 1941;32:189–199.
11 Downey M, Hickey BB, Sharp ME: The acid phosphatase content of the enlarged and malignant prostate gland with some observations on histopathology as revealed by Gomori's staining. Br J Urol 1954;26:160–165.
12 Parkin L, Bylsma G, Torre AV, Drew D, Madden RJ: Acid phosphatase in carcinoma of the prostate in man. J Histochem Cytochem 1964; 12:288–292.

13 Shulman S, Manrod L, Gonder M, Soanes WA: The detection of prostatic acid phosphatase by antibody reactions in gel diffusions. J Immunol 1964;93:474–480.
14 Gutman AB: The development of the acid phosphatase test for prostatic carcinoma. Bull NY Acad Med 1968;44:63–76.
15 Wang MC, Valenzuela CA, Murphy GP, Chu TM: Purification of a human prostate specific antigen. Invest Urol 1979;17:159–163.
16 Sinha AA, Gleason DF, Wilson MJ, Wick MR, Reddy PK, Blackard CE: Relationship of prostatic acid phosphatase localization in human prostate by a monoclonal antibody with the Gleason grading system. Prostate 1988;13:1–15.
17 Warhol MJ, Longtine JA: The ultrastructural localization of prostatic specific antigen and prostatic acid phosphatase in hyperplastic and neoplastic human prostates. J Urol 1985;134: 607–613.
18 Sinha AA, Wilson MJ, Gleason DF: Immunoelectron microscopic localization of prostatic-specific antigen in human prostate by the protein A-gold complex. Cancer 1987;60: 1288–1293.
19 Bates RJ, Chapman CM, Prout GR Jr, Lin CW: Immunohistochemical identification of prostatic acid phosphatase: Correlation of tumor grade with acid phosphatase distribution. J Urol 1982;127:574–580.
20 Benz MS, Cohen C, Demers LM, Budgeon LR: Immunohistochemical acid phosphatase level and tumor grade in prostatic cancer. Arch Pathol Lab Med 1982;106:476–480.
21 Stein BS, Petersen RO, Vangore S, Kendall AR: Immunoperoxidase localization of prostate-specific antigen. Am J Surg Pathol 1982;6: 553–557.
22 Shevchuk MM, Romas NA, Ying PO, Tannenbaum M, Olsson CA: Acid phosphatase localization in prostatic carcinoma. A comparison of monoclonal antibody to heteroantisera. Cancer 1983;52:1642–1646.
23 Epstein JI, Eggleston JC: Immunohistochemical localization of prostate-specific acid phosphatase and prostate-specific antigen in stage $A_2$ adenocarcinoma of the prostate: Prognostic implications. Hum Pathol 1984;15:853–859.
24 Feiner HD, Gonzales R: Carcinoma of the prostata with atypical immunohistological features. Clinical and histologic correlates. Am J Surg Pathol 1986;10:765–770.
25 Nadji M, Tabei SZ, Castro A, Chu TM, Morales AR: Prostatic origin of tumors. An immunohistochemical study. Am J Clin Pathol 1980; 73:735–739.
26 Walker AN, Mills SE, Fechner RE, Perry JM: 'Endometrial' adenocarcinoma of the prostatic urethra arising in a villous polyp. A light microscopic and immunoperoxidase study. Arch Pathol Lab Med 1982;106:624–627.
27 Bostwick DG, Kindrachuk RW, Rouse RV: Prostatic adenocarcinoma with endometrioid features. Clinical, pathologic, and ultrastructural findings. Am J Surg Pathol 1985;9:595–609.
28 Epstein JI, Woodruff JM: Adenocarcinoma of the prostate with endometrioid features. A light microscopic and immunohistochemical study of ten cases. Cancer 1986;57:111–119.
29 Wernert N, Lüchtrath H, Seelinger H, Schäfer M, Goebbels R, Dhom G: Papillary carcinoma of the prostate, location, morphology, and immunohistochemistry: The histogenesis and entity of so-called endometrioid carcinoma. Prostate 1987;10:123–131.
30 Jöbsis AC, De Vries GP, Anholt RRH, Sanders GTB: Demonstration of the prostatic origin of metastases. An immunohistochemical method for formalin-fixed embedded tissue. Cancer 1978;41:1788–1793.
31 Nadji M, Tabei SZ, Castro A, Chu TM, Murphy GP, Wang MC, Morales AR: Prostatic-specific antigen. An immunohistologic marker for prostatic neoplasms. Cancer 1981;48:1229–1232.
32 Stein BS, Vangore S, Petersen RO: Immunoperoxidase localization of prostatic antigens. Comparison of primary and metastatic sites. Urology 1984;24:146–152.
33 Grignon D, Troster M: Changes in immunohistochemical staining in prostatic adenocarcinoma following diethylstilbestrol therapy. Prostate 1985;7:195–202.
34 Têtu B, Srigley JR, Boivin J-C, Dupont A, Monfette G, Pinault S, Labrie F: Effect of combination endocrine therapy (LHRH agonist and flutamide) on normal prostate and prostatic adenocarcinoma. Am J Surg Pathol 1991; 15:111–120.
35 Cohen C, Bentz MS, Budgeon LR: Prostatic acid phosphatase in carcinoid and islet cell tumours (letter). Arch Pathol Lab Med 1983; 107:277.
36 Yam LT, Jackila AJ, Lam WKW, Li CY: Immunohistochemistry of prostatic acid phosphatase. Prostate 1981;2:97–107.
37 Kimura N, Sasano N: Prostate-specific acid phosphatase in carcinoid tumors. Virchows Arch [A] 1986;410:247–251.
38 Azumi N, Traweek ST, Battifora H: Prostatic acid phosphatase in carcinoid tumors. Immunohistochemical and immunoblot studies. Am J Surg Pathol 1991;15:785–790.
39 Epstein JI, Kuhajda FP, Lieberman PH: Prostate-specific acid phosphatase immunoreactivity in adenocarcinomas of the urinary bladder. Hum Pathol 1986;17:939–942.
40 Papotti M, Paties C, Peveri V, Moscuzza L, Bussolati G: Immunocytochemical detection of prostate-specific antigen in skin adnexal and breast tissues and tumors. Basic Appl Histochem 1989;33:25–29.
41 Moll R, Franke WW; Schiller DL, Geiger B, Krepler R: The catalogue of human cytokeratin polypeptides: Patterns of expression of specific cytokeratins in normal epithelia, tumors and cultured cells. Cell 1982;31:11–24.
42 Kuwahara T, Nagayama T: Distribution of keratin protein in normal prostate and prostatic tumors. An immunohistochemical study. Acta Pathol Jpn 1987;37:339–342.
43 Nagle RB, Ahmann FR, McDaniel KM, Paquin ML, Clark VA, Celniker A: Cytokeratin characterization of human prostatic carcinoma and its derived cell lines. Cancer Res 1987;47: 281–286.
44 Wernert N, Seitz G, Achtstatter T: Immunohistochemical investigation of different cytokeratins and vimentin in the prostate from the fetal period up to adulthood and in prostate carcinoma. Pathol Res Pract 1987;182:617–626.
45 Bostwick DG, Brawer MK: Prostatic intra-epithelial neoplasia and early invasion in prostate cancer. Cancer 1987;59:788–794.
46 Grignon DJ, Ro JY, Ordônez NG, Ayala AG, Cleary KR: Basal cell hyperplasia, adenoid basal cell tumor, and adenoid cystic carcinoma of the prostate gland: An immunohistochemical study. Hum Pathol 1988;19:1425–1433.
47 Nagle RB, Brawer MK, Kittelson J, Clark V: Phenotypic relationship of prostatic intraepithelial neoplasia to invasive prostatic carcinoma. Am J Pathol 1991;138:119–128.
48 Abrahamsson P-A, Waldström LB, Alumets J, Falkmer S, Grimelius L: Peptide-hormone- and serotonin-immunoreactive tumour cells in carcinoma of the prostate. Pathol Res Pract 1987;182:298–307.
49 di Sant'Agnese PA, De Mesi Jensen KL: Neuroendocrine differentiation in prostatic carcinoma. Hum Pathol 1987;18:849–856.
50 Turbet-Herrera EA, Herrera GA, Gore I, Lott RL, Grizzle WE, Bonnin JM: Neuroendocrine differentiation in prostatic carcinomas. A retrospective autopsy study. Arch Pathol Lab Med 1988;112:1100–1105.
51 Têtu B, Ro JY, Ayala AG, Johnson DE, Logothetis CJ, Ordonez NG: Small cell carcinoma of the prostate. I. A clinicopathologic study of 20 cases. Cancer 1987;59:1803–1809.
52 Ro JY, Têtu B, Ayala AG, Ordonez NG: Small cell carcinoma of the prostate. II. Immunohistochemical and electron microscopic studies of 18 cases. Cancer 1987;59:977–982.
53 Hagood PG, Johnson FE, Bedrossian CWM, Silverberg AB: Small cell carcinoma of the prostate. Cancer 1991;67:1046–1050.
54 Azumi N, Shibuya H, Ishikura M: Primary prostatic carcinoid tumor with intracytoplasmic prostatic acid phosphatase and prostate-specific antigen. Am J Surg Pathol 1984;8:545–550.
55 Abrahamsson P-A, Falkmer S, Falt K, Grimelius L: The course of neuroendocrine differentiation in prostatic carcinomas. An immunohistochemical study testing chromogranin A as an 'endocrine marker'. Pathol Res Pract 1989; 185:373–380.
56 di Sant'Agnese PA: Neuroendocrine differentiation and prostatic carcinoma. The concept 'comes of age'. Arch Pathol Lab Med 1988;112: 1097–1099.
57 McNeal JE, Alroy J, Leav I, Redwine EA, Freiha FS, Stamey TA: Immunohistochemical evidence for impaired cell differentiation in the premalignant phase of prostate carcinogenesis. Am J Clin Pathol 1988;90:23–32.
58 Chastonay P, Hurlimann J, Gardiol D: Biological tissue markers in benign and malignant disease of the human prostate. Virchows Arch [A] 1986;410:221–229.
59 Walker PD, Karnik S, deKernion JB, Pramberg JC: Cell surface blood group antigens in prostatic carcinoma. Am J Clin Pathol 1984; 81:503–506.

Eur Urol 1992;21(suppl 1):71–74

*P. Marandola*[a], *B. Lardennois*[b]
*D. Ploton*[b], *M. Derenzini*[c]
*D. Treré*[c], *B. Campo*[a]
*P. Corrada*[a], *V. Valentino*[a]
*A. Roggia*[a], *P. Broggini*[a]
*D. Vicini*[a], *G.P. Franceschetti*[a]
*C. Iweha*[a], *A. Speroni*[a]

[a] School of Urology, University of Pavia, Italy;
[b] CHRU, Reims, France, and
[c] University of Bologna, Italy

# Nucleolar Organizer Regions: Preliminary Results of the Clinical Use of a New Marker for Prostatic Carcinoma (40 Cases)

**Key Words**
Prostate
Prognostic factors
Nucleolar organizer regions

**Abstract**
It is a widely diffused opinion that moving backwards in time the moment of the diagnosis of cancer of prostate, so that the tumor is detected earlier than normal, means that the treatment would be more effective than the one adopted in the usual times of diagnosis. For this reason the earlier diagnosis of prostate cancer has become more and more a compulsory target of the modern urologist, at a time of booming of the third age, of increased lifetime expectancy, of significant elevation of prostate cancer rate and of the persistent uncertainty of the efficacy of available treatments. Theoretically the mortality rate of prostate cancer can be reduced by the prevention programs and by the improvements of treatment methods, but the 'earlier' diagnosis is certainly an easier and less expensive strategy to achieve the same objective. The authors have evaluated the argyrophilic-nucleolar organizer region (Ag-NOR) proteins on 40 cases of adenocarcinoma of prostate collected through a multicentric program in France and in Italy. The Ag-NOR have been stained with silver technique set up by Ploton and Derenzini while the quantitative index has been evaluated by a semiautomatic system partially commercially available, partially modified by the authors. The conclusions: (a) the Ag-NOR index is a simple and reproducible method; (b) the Ag-NOR staging system corresponds to Gleason's grading; (c) the Ag-NOR elevation is a reliable marker of increased cell proliferation and is detectable much earlier than the morphologic changes of Gleason's classification.

## Introduction

The natural history of prostatic carcinoma is characterized by a long latency period before its clinical appearance, rendering imperative the need to study diagnostic and prognostic factors capable of demonstrating the presence of cancer and its classification before its clinical and symptomatic debut [9, 10]. It is well known that treatment results are better when the diagnosis and therapeutic modalities are taken backwards in the time before the natural history of the cancer, especially if a certain quality of life for the patient with prostate cancer is to be preserved.

Presently the diagnostic methods in use are late morphological indicators of tumor insurgence; changes in biohumoral parameters appear late in the disease and are therefore of little use; sonographic evidence is often late

Prof. Paolo Marandola
School of Urology, University of Pavia
Policlinico S. Matteo
I-27100 Pavia (Italy)


0302–2838/92/0215–0071
$2.75/0

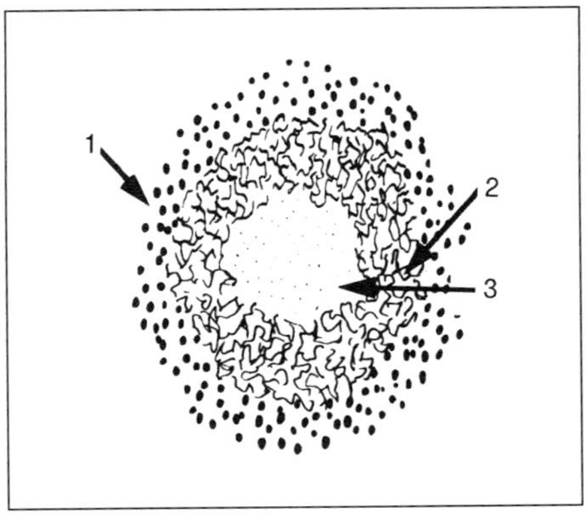


**Fig. 1.** NOR ultrastructure (interface): 1 = granular component; Z = dense fibrillary component; 3 = fibrillary center.

and dubious and depend on the operator's ability; biopsy and the relative histological diagnosis are less objective methodologies [8–11]. The attention to subcellular parameters can be useful in the evaluation of the evolution of neoplastic lesions (fig. 1).

Tumor cells are constantly showing morphological nucleolar modifications, consisting in an increase and deformation of nucleolar size. The study of these structures must be done with appropriate methods so as to obtain objective results.

Recent studies on the ultrastructural morphology have shown that the size and form of the nucleoli are a consequence of the number and distribution of definite nucleolar components bearing the genes synthesizing ribosomal RNA. These structures are commonly defined nucleolar organizer regions (NORs) visible in interphase nuclei from the term used by cytogenetists to indicate those areas of secondary constrictions which in metaphasic chromosomes contain ribosomal coding genes. Geossens [7] demonstrated that argyrophilia is due to the presence of nonhistonic proteins (Ag-NOR) which regulates the activity of DNAr and that the intensity of the argyrophilia is directly proportional to the transcriptional activity of the nucleolus [6, 14, 15]. These observations became important when Ploton and co-workers [12, 13] developed a cytohistologic method based on colloid silver staining which selectively visualizes the Ag-NORs, visible at the optic microscope or the electron microscope. These Ag-NOR proteins precipitate metallic silver upon contact with the colloid silver solution.

This technique has been extended to preparations in paraffin, which allows the precipitation of silver nitrate on acidic proteins corresponding to NORs if pretreated with Carnoy. NORs appear as separate black dots within a pale yellow-colored nucleus. Both the time and the coloring techniques, the method and types of fixative are under study; a corrective parameter which will enable a comparison of the results obtained using a different method is being defined. The observation obtained from different types of benign and malignant tumors, equipped with quantitative and semiquantitative analyses, have demonstrated the possibility of easily distinguishing benign from malignant cells according to the increase in the number of Ag-NORs, and according to their irregular distribution within the nucleoli [4, 5].

It will be possible to make prognostic considerations reading NORs within the frame of borderline neoplastic lesions and slowly growing lesions. A parameter with such diagnosis and prognostic characteristics should be above subjective considerations or evaluations [1, 2]. To this end, a semiautomatic system has been studied for reading and evaluating NORs. Such a system is composed of an image analyzer fitted with the appropriate software. The choice of an appropriate phase of nucleoli for measurement, in the absence of artifacts, is a sufficiently good focus done manually with a pointer for an optimal interpretation. The technique consists of a mean evaluation of 100 nuclei, which requires about 5 min and is therefore possible in routine practice.

Single values could be shown using graphs that highlight their homogeneous nature. The results of our initial experience based only on retrospective considerations were not optimal; due to difficulties inherent in reading paraffin-embedded sections, they show a correlation between the value of NOR and the neoplastic grade at the time of diagnosis, besides, a notable correlation has been observed between the value of NOR and tumor evolution.

## Materials and Methods

A retrospective study was carried out on a sample of 40 selected patients with cancer of the prostate. The first segment was initiated in Reims in 1978 by Lardennois and Ploton with two groups of patients with advanced cancer of the prostate. The second segment was initiated in Pavia and Bologna in 1990 but the criteria for patient selection have been the same for both groups. The same methodologies have been used for the measurement of NOR activity in both segments of the study. The patient population has been heterogeneous for age, stage of the disease and treatment protocols. The criteria used have been those of TNM classification, other clinical indicators and the quality of life of the patients in the environment; the absence of metastasis at the time of diagnosis and PAP $< 10$ IU. Patients who benefitted from a curative treatment were excluded from the program because that could have modified the natural progression of the disease [3].

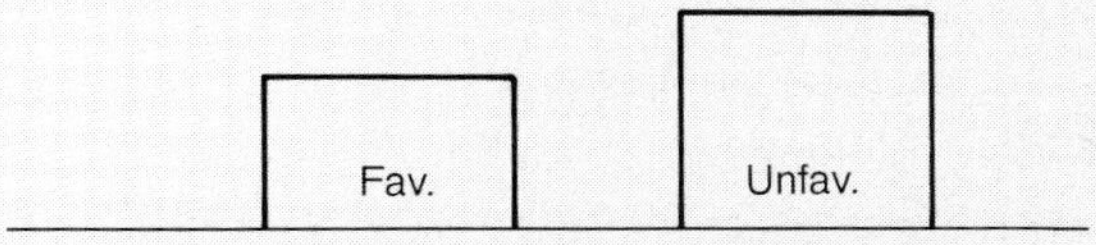


| NOR | Fav. | Unfav. |
|---|---|---|
| Number | 21 | 17 |
| Mean | 7.00 | 9.97 |
| SD | 2.35 | 2.63 |

t = 2.43 ⟶ p < 0.02 (significant)

2

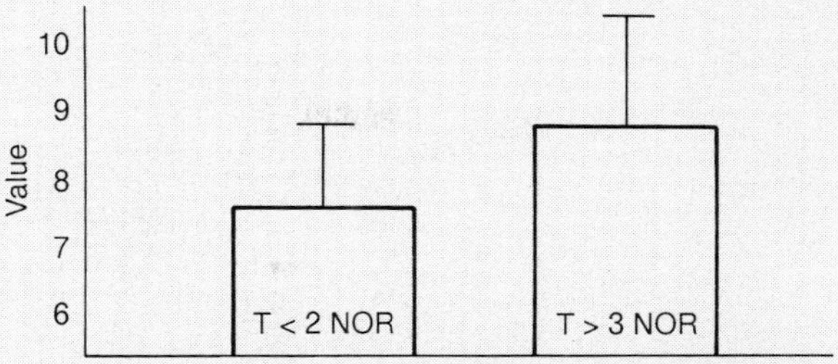


| | NOR < or = 2 | NOR > or = 3 |
|---|---|---|
| Number | 21 | 17 |
| Mean | 7.48 | 8.35 |
| SD | 2.82 | 2.42 |

t = 1.004 ⟶ p = NS

3

**Fig. 2.** Comparison of NOR favorable/unfavorable evolution.

**Fig. 3.** Comparison of T $<2$ NOR and T $>3$ NOR. All evolutions are mixed up.

Two patient groups were chosen without considering the initial T: one group with a favorable evolution (21 patients) and another with an unfavorable evolution (19 patients). The two groups were statistically comparable, without metastasis and homogeneous as regards tumor grade. Tumor evolution was defined not only in terms of the quantity but also on the quality of survival. A good correlation of NOR with the prognosis seems to indicate that the method could have an important impact in deciding the treatment modality.

As in every retrospective study there were difficulties: data not being collected by the same person with the same follow-up protocol, reliability of certain exams, e.g. digital rectal exploration, the interpretation of tumor size varies among clinicians.

The aim of this study is to correlate the value of NOR with the prognosis of carcinoma and therefore with the evolution of the disease in relation with the initial T, with the value of NOR after visual and automatic lecture and with the Gleason index. NOR values for normal prostate have been compared with NOR values for neoplastic prostate, where 'normal' prostate corresponds to nonneoplastic prostate tissue taken from five different sections of our sample. NOR activity is determined and compared to the NOR activity of the neoplastic prostate tissue. The variations of NOR values of the favorable group have been compared to those of the unfavorable group. The variations of the NOR index with the initial T, e.g. T $<2$, T $>3$, have been compared without considering their evolutions. NOR-Gleason correlations have been studied comparing their respective predictive values for each group of patients.

## Results

We had 40 pairs of microscopic slides for the two lecture methods: visual and semiautomatic, and the results obtained with a margin of correction of 95%. We have compared the 21 NOR values of patients with a favorable evolution with the 19 of unfavorable evolution. The mean NOR value for the group with favorable evolution is 7.00 with a deviation of 2.35 while that of the unfavorable evolution is 8.97 with a deviation of 2.63 (fig. 2). Student's test gives t = 2.43. There is a significant difference between the NOR values of both groups, the values are higher for the group with the unfavorable evolution and the margin of error is less than 2% ($p < 0.02$). For the 'normal' prostate sample, the mean NOR index is 2.87 with a deviation of 0.43 while the mean NOR index for neoplastic prostate tissue is 6.87 with a deviation of 2.99. Student's test allows t = 2.957. This gives a significant difference between the two series of NOR indices with a margin of error of less than 1% ($p < 0.01$). The comparison is between the NOR index and the primitive tumor volume: 21 patients had T $<2$ and 19 had T $>3$. For the group with T $<2$, the mean NOR value is 7.48 with a deviation of 2.82; for the group with T $>3$ it is 8.35 with a deviation of 2.42. Student's test shows t = 1.004 (fig. 3). The difference in NOR values is not significant for the tumor volume of both groups.

When NOR values are compared to the Gleason index we were able to obtain a coefficient of correlation = 0.30. There is a positive significance for this sample and for predictive methods ($p = 0.02$).

## Discussion

We have used Student's test on the assumption that our samples approximately followed the gaussian curve together with our biological data. The samples were

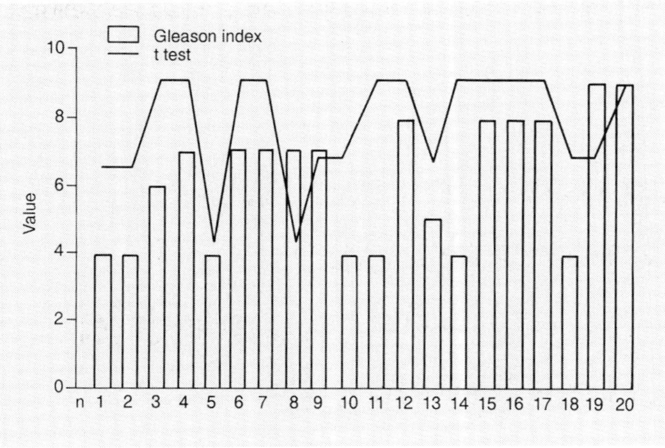


**Fig. 4.** Comparative t test and Gleason index.

obtained from virgin prostate tissue, i.e. without prior treatment from diagnostic material. Treatment programs were identified for each patient and palliative treatments have little influence on survival.

We have been able to show that the tumors with unfavorable evolution had a significantly higher NOR index at the time of diagnosis than those with a favorable evolution. After having considered the performance of all classical prognostic markers, both morphologic and biohumoral of prostate cancer, we have not much information available for the cure of the patient with prostate cancer. It is our opinion that the prognosis for the cancer of the prostate cannot be determined only by histology. The cytologic grade and the Gleason index are presently our only advantage, but unfortunately there are many regarding intermediate grades and borderline lesions (fig. 4). With the NOR index we think we have a simple and reliable method of appraising the activity and therefore the aggressivity of tumors. The NOR index is an index of cell proliferation obtainable through microscopic intranucleolar lecture. These numerical values are reproducible and applied on carefully selected 40 patients with prostate cancer. We have been able to define the evolution profile of the disease for each patient by trying to determine 'favorable' or 'unfavorable'. Despite the difficulties inherent with the readings, the statistical methods used have allowed us to demonstrate that among the two groups there was a significant difference between the initial NOR values; that the variation in NOR index is not parallel with tumor volume; that tumor progression in terms of duration of survival is correlated with the NOR index. We can say that the predictive value of NOR index has been good.

A prospective study is underway for a reconsideration of data obtained from optimal sections from a technical point of view, only after a few years can we obtain a confirmation of the effective value of this new parameter. High NOR indices will in principle orientate towards an aggressive therapeutic behavior on the part of the urologist, while a low NOR index will indicate a more conservative approach.

## References


1 Adnet JJ: Les organisateurs nucléolaires: intérêt en anatomie pathologique et en cytologie clinique. Ann Pathol 1989;9:3–6.

2 Adnet JJ, Ploton D, Pinteaux A, Lecki C: Les organisateurs nucléolaires en pathologie tumorale. 69 ème Congrès de l'Association des Anatomistes. Bull Assoc Anat 1987;71:213–219.

3 Byar DP, Mostofi FK: Carcinoma of the prostate: prognostic evaluation of certain pathologic features in 208 radical prostatectomies examined by the ste-section technique. Cancer 1972;30:5.

4 Colloby PS, Crocker J: Nucleolar organizer regions in prostatic malignancy; in Underwood JCE (ed): Current Topics in Pathology. Pathology of the Nucleus. New York, Springer, 1990, p 135.

5 Crocker J: Nucleolar organizer regions; in Underwood JCE (ed): Current Topics in Pathology. Pathology of the Nucleus. New York, Springer, 1990, pp 92–149.

6 Egan M, Raafat F, Crocker J, Williams D: Comparative study of the degree of differentiation of neuroblastoma and mean numbers of nucleolar organizer regions. J Clin Pathol 1988; 41:527–531.

7 Geossens G: Nucleolar structure. Int Rev Cytol 1984;87:107–158.

8 Gleason DF, Mellinger GT, and the Veterans Administration Cooperative Urological Research Group: Prediction of prognosis for prostatic adenocarcinoma by combined histological grading and clinical staging. J Urol 1974;111: 58.

9 McNeal JE, Bostwick DG, Kindrauchuck RA, Redwine EA, Freiha FS, Stamey TA: Patterns of progression in prostate cancer. Lancet 1986; i:60.

10 McNeal JE: Origin and development of carcinoma in the prostate. Cancer 1969;23:24.

11 Mostofi FK, Davis CJ, Sesterhenn IA: Pathology of tumors of the urinary tract; in Skinner DG, Lieskovski G (eds): Diagnosis and Management of Genitourinary Cancer. Philadelphia, Saunders, 1988, pp 83–117.

12 Ploton D: Etude de la localisation des protéines nucléolaires argyrophiles dans les cellules cancéreuses humaines interphasiques et mitotiques; thesis Paris 1988.

13 Ploton D, Menager M, Jeanesson P: Improvement in the staining and in the visualization of the Ag-NOR protein (argyrophilic proteins of the nucleolar organizer region) at the optical level. Histochem J 1985;18:5–14.

14 Trere D, Pession A, Derenzini M: The silver stained proteins of interphasic nucleolar organizer regions as a parameter of cell duplication rate. Exp Cell Res 1989;184:131–139.

15 Vazeux H: Les organisateurs nucléolaires (NOR): nouvel indicateur prognostique du cancer de la prostate; thesis Reims 1990.

Eur Urol 1992;21 (suppl 1):75–78

*F. Clar-Blanch*[a]
*L. Morell-Quadreny*[b]
*B. Fenollosa-Entrena*[c]
*P. Chuan-Nuez*[a]
*M. Gil-Salom*[a]
*P. Carretero-Gonzalez*[a]
*A. Llombart-Bosch*[b]

[a] Service of Urology, Hospital Clínico Universitario, Valencia;
[b] Department of Pathology, University of Valencia, and
[c] Service of Preventive Medicine, Hospital La Fe, Valencia, Spain

# Correlation between Serum Values of Prostatic Acid Phosphatase and Morphometric Analysis in the Cytologic Diagnosis of Prostatic Carcinoma

**Key Words**
Prostatic acid phosphatase
Morphometry analysis
Cytology
Prostatic carcinoma

**Abstract**
We studied 78 men with suspicion of prostatic carcinoma, who underwent transrectal aspiration biopsy, diagnosing 46 adenocarcinoma, 13 chronic prostatitis and 19 benign prostatic hyperplasia. Moreover, we determined prostatic acid phosphatase (PAP) by enzyme immunoanalysis, resulting in 9/78 false-positives and 18/78 false-negatives. Also, we carried out a morphometric analysis of the cytologic samples which showed good correlation with the cytologic diagnosis except in the moderately differentiated carcinomas. We found a good correlation between PAP values, cytologic diagnosis and nuclear size as well as the percentage of the binucleolated cells.

Acid phosphatase was the first substance to be used in human pathology as a tumor marker. Bodansky [1] in 1933, Gutman and Gutman [2] in 1938, and Huggins and Hodges [3] in 1941, were the first authors to appreciate its increase in the serum of patients suffering from metastatic prostatic adenocarcinoma, as well as its subsequent diminution as a result of the hormonal treatment.

From that time onwards it has been widely used as a tumor marker in prostatic adenocarcinoma. In 1960, Flocks et al. [4] isolated antibodies against the human prostatic tissue, thus creating the first immunologic methods in the determination of acid phosphatase. In 1964, Shulman et al. [5] described prostatic acid phosphatase (PAP) as the specific prostatic antigen, thus allowing the development of several immunologic methods, such as the determination through enzyme immunoanalysis (EIA), which showed advantages over the traditional enzymatic methods [6].

There is a correlation between the production of acid phosphatase, the histological degree and the aggressiveness of the tumor [7]. As regards the prognosis of the prostatic cancer, it is difficult to establish it with certainty at an individual level. One of the proposed techniques, the one which seems to correlate best with survival, is the morphometric and stereologic analysis of nuclei and nucleoli from prostatic carcinoma cells [8, 9].

## Patients and Methods

We performed a prospective study on a group of 78 men who were clinically suspicious of having prostatic carcinoma. Their PAP was determined by means of EIA with monoclonal antibodies. Pathologic diagnosis was done with a puncture aspiration with a Franzen needle. Morphometric analyses were made with a Zeiss-Konton, model MOP Videoplan 2,000, on the cytologic preparations. 200 cellular nuclei were measured each time while determining

Dr. Francisco Clar-Blanch
Service of Urology, Hospital Clinico Universitario
C/. Guardia Civil 7, 3° C
E-46020 Valencia (Spain)


0302–2838/92/0215–0075
$2.75/0

their area, perimeter, and maximum nuclear diameter. The shape factor was stereologically determined. Moreover, in 31 cases, 100 nucleoli were measured with the same equipment, determining not only their area, perimeter and maximum diameter, but also the percentage of bi-, tri-, and multinucleolated cells. The statistical part of the study was done with a Hewlett-Packard 9825-A computer, programme series 200-PP.

**Table 1**

| | | CTAN | CTPN | CTDM | CTFE |
|---|---|---|---|---|---|
| Poor. diff. | $\bar{x}$ | 65.5 | 29.6 | 9.99 | 0.85 |
| | SD | 17.6 | 4.15 | 1.36 | 0.01 |
| | n | 7 | 7 | 7 | 7 |
| Mod. diff. | $\bar{x}$ | 43.0 | 23.9 | 8.17 | 0.86 |
| | SD | 11.0 | 3.06 | 0.99 | 0.02 |
| | n | 18 | 18 | 18 | 18 |
| Well diff. | $\bar{x}$ | 45.6 | 24.7 | 8.25 | 0.85 |
| | SD | 11.5 | 3.04 | 1.07 | 0.03 |
| | n | 21 | 21 | 21 | 21 |
| Chronic p. | $\bar{x}$ | 29.6 | 20.5 | 6.61 | 0.87 |
| | SD | 7.01 | 3.81 | 0.75 | 0.02 |
| | n | 13 | 13 | 13 | 13 |
| BHP | $\bar{x}$ | 29.4 | 19.9 | 6.68 | 0.86 |
| | SD | 4.58 | 1.63 | 0.60 | 0.02 |
| | n | 18 | 18 | 18 | 18 |

CTAN = nuclear area; CTPN = nuclear perimeter; CTDM = maximum diameter nuclear; CTFE: stereologic shape factor.
$\bar{x}$ = Average; SD = standard deviation; n = cases.

**Table 2**

| | | CTan | CTbn | CTtn | CTmn |
|---|---|---|---|---|---|
| Poor diff. | $\bar{x}$ | 3.69 | 11.7 | 8.11 | 3.15 |
| | SD | 1.13 | 5.69 | 6.69 | 3.05 |
| | n | 4 | 4 | 4 | 4 |
| Mod. diff. | $\bar{x}$ | 3.23 | 13.1 | 3.71 | 0.32 |
| | SD | 0.99 | 8.06 | 3.68 | 0.65 |
| | n | 13 | 13 | 13 | 13 |
| Well diff. | $\bar{x}$ | 2.32 | 9.47 | 1.22 | 0.07 |
| | SD | 0.67 | 4.43 | 1.69 | 0.27 |
| | n | 14 | 14 | 14 | 14 |

CTan = nucleolar area of mononucleolated cells; CTbn = percentage of binucleolated cells; CTtn = percentage of trinucleolated cells; CTmn = percentage of multinucleolated cells.
$\bar{x}$ = Average; SD = standard deviation; n = cases.

## Results

Of the 78 patients studied, 46 were adenocarcinomas, 13 chronic prostatitis and 19 benign prostatic hyperplasia; all had been diagnosed by means of transrectal aspiration biopsy. The determination of PAP was as expected in 51 cases, whereas it was false-positive in 9 cases (11.53%) and false-negative in 18 cases (23.07%). The morphometric analysis showed that the nuclear areas of the cancer samples were larger than those of benign pathology (chronic prostatitis and benign prostatic hyperplasia), with differences that were statistically significant, although these differences were neither evident among the different types of cancer nor between chronic prostatitis and benign prostatic hyperplasia (table 1).

In mononucleolated cells we observed a medium value of the nucleolar area that is higher in poorly differentiated carcinomas, as well as a higher standard deviation. These values decrease as the tumor becomes increasingly differentiated (table 2).

In those tumors whose cells presented more than one nucleolus, the percentage of bi-, tri-, and multinucleolated cells has been determined. It has been observed that moderately differentiated tumors presented a higher percentage of binucleolated cells, whereas those that were well differentiated presented this type of cell less often. The higher percentage of trinucleolated cells corresponded to the tumors that were poorly differentiated and it diminished progressively in correlation to the greater differentiation of the tumor.

The cytologic diagnosis has presented a significant statistical relationship with PAP determined by EIA ($p < 0.05$). PAP clearly distinguished cancer from benign prostatic hyperplasia ($p < 0.05$) whereas it did not in the case of cancer and chronic prostatitis. Significant differences were equally observed between PAP and the values of the nuclear area ($p < 0.05$), maximum nuclear diameter ($p < 0.05$), and the percentage of binucleolated cells ($p < 0.05$).

## Discussion

In our investigation, 9 patients were considered false-positive, which made a total of 11.53%. Four out of these 9 were diagnosed as chronic prostatitis, and 5 as benign prostatic hyperplasia. It must be mentioned that all the patients suffering from hyperplasia wore a urethral catheter permanently, which, according to Griffiths et al. [10] and Bruce et al. [11] is sufficient to elevate the PAP. Our results are better than those obtained by Oosterom et al. [12], who detected 17% false-positives. The higher the amount of PAP, the lower the number of false-positives. When the PAP reaches 10.0 ng/ml (5 times over the average) we discover no false-positives. False-negatives amounted to 18 (23.07%), out of whom 13 suffered from a localized and 5 from a metastatic adenocarcinoma. These results can be compared to those of other authors [12, 13].

The morphometric study of cells obtained by transrectal aspiration biopsy showed statistically significant differences between the benign and the malignant cells in their areas, perimeters and maximum diameters. However, morphometry did not show a clear difference between chronic prostatitis and hyperplasia; neither could it divide carcinomas according to their degree of tumoral differentiation with statistically significant differences. Such differences were only observed in poorly differentiated carcinomas, with measures of size and standard deviation, which were higher than in the other 2 cases. This corroborates the observations of most authors who consider that these tumors belong to the category of those poorly differentiated [14–16]. Moreover, morphometric results related to the nucleolar area have clearly distinguished between the highly differentiated carcinoma and the other two. This reveals the importance of the nucleoli for the evaluation of the prostatic pathology [16–18].

As regards the percentage of multinucleolated cells present in the smears, we observe that poorly differentiated carcinomas, when compared with those that are well differentiated, exceed such a percentage with statistically significant differences, both when cells are trinucleolated and when they have more than three nucleoli. Besides, moderately differentiated carcinomas occupy an intermediate position between the two, with no significant differences in the percentage of trinucleolated cells. They only reveal differences in the percentage of multinucleolated cells when compared with the poorly differentiated carcinoma. Our results equal those of Helpap [17], who observes that the higher the degree of malignancy, the higher the number of nucleoli in the prostatic carcinoma. Therefore, moderately differentiated tumors deserve special attention for, although they resemble well-differentiated tumors in their nuclear size, their nucleolar activity resembles that of poorly differentiated ones.

As regards tumor markers, the nucleolar area has a statistically significant relationship ($p < 0.05$) with PAP. The latter is, at the same time, related to the percentage of binucleolated cells ($p < 0.05$), which does not occur in the case of cells with three nucleoli or more. This would corroborate what Pontes et al. [19] and Lange and Winfield [20] said when pointing out that cells, when becoming anaplastic, so increasing, as we have seen, the number of nucleoli, cease to synthesize acid phosphatase. Other authors [21] admit the possibility that the negativity of acid phosphatase in prostatic carcinomas be due to the heterogeneity of the tumor since there exist cancerous cells which do not produce acid phosphatase.

On the evidence of our results we cannot establish any biochemical-morphometric correlation which implies a certain prognosis. To conclude, we must say that if morphometry cannot separate the different degrees of tumoral differentiation, it may be due to the fact that they be inseparable, for – as Baak [22] indicates – they belong to a continuous spectrum whose limits are not easy to define, not even – as has been the case here – with more objective means than the pathologist's eye. However, this stimulates us to follow these patients closely, in the hope that in the future all these data that cannot be fully worked out may throw some light on the evolution of these patients.

## References


1 Bodansky A: Phosphatase studies. II. Determination of serum phosphatase. Factors influencing the accuracy of the determination. J Biol Chem 1933;101:93–105.

2 Gutman AB, Gutman EB: 'Acid' phosphatase occurring in the serum of patients with metastasizing carcinoma of the prostate gland. J Clin Invest 1938;17:473–478.

3 Huggins C, Hodges CV: Studies on prostatic cancer. The effects of castration of estrogen and of androgen injection on serum phosphatases in metastatic carcinoma of the prostate. Cancer Res 1941;1:293–297.

4 Flocks RH, Urich VC, Patel CA, Opith JM: Studies on the antigenic properties of prostatic tissue. J Urol 1960;84:134–143.

5 Shulman S, Mamrod L, Gonder MJ, Soanes WA: The detection of prostatic acid phosphatase by antibody reactions in gel diffusion. J Immunol 1964;93:474–480.

6 Choe BK, Rose NR, Korol M: Immunoenzyme assay for human prostatic acid phosphatase. Proc Soc Exp Biol Med 1979;162:396–398.

7 Bates RJ, Chapman CM, Prout GR Jr, Ling CW: Immunohistochemical identification of prostatic acid phosphatase: correlation of tumor grade with acid phosphatase distribution. J Urol 1982;127:574–580.

8 Diamond DA, Berry SJ, Jewett HJ, Eggleston JC, Coffey DS: A new method to assess metastatic potential of human prostatic cancer: Relative nuclear roundness. J Urol 1982;128:729–734.

9 Tannenbaum M, Tannenbaum S, De Sanctis P, Olson C: Prognostic significance of nucleolar surface area in prostatic cancer. Urology 1982; 5:546–551.

10 Griffiths J, Rippe DF; Panfili PR: Comparison of enzyme-linked immunoadsorbent assay and radioimmunoassay for prostate-specific acid phosphatase in prostatic disease. Clin Chem 1982;28:183–186.
11 Bruce AW, Mahan DE, Sullivan LD, Goldenberg L: The significance of prostatic acid phosphatase in adenocarcinoma of the prostate. J Urol 1981;125:357–360.
12 Oosterom R, Leijnse B, Bogdanowicz J, Schroeder FH: Evaluation of an enzyme immunoassay for prostatic acid phosphatase utilizing monoclonal antibodies. Worl J Urol 1986;4: 153–158.
13 Kuriyama M, Wang MC, Lee CL: Multiple marker evaluation in human prostate cancer with the use of tissue-specific antigens. J Natl Cancer Inst 1982;68:99–104.
14 Esposti PL: Cytologic malignancy grading of prostatic carcinoma by transrectal aspiration biopsy. Scand J Urol Nephrol 1971;5:199–209.
15 Leistenschneider W, Nagel R: Atlas of Prostatic Cytology. Techniques and Diagnosis. Berlin, Springer 1984.
16 Koss LG, Woyke S, Olszeewski W: Prostata; in Biopsia por aspiración. Interpretación citológica y bases histológicas. Buenos Aires, Ed Panamericana, 1988, pp 251–276.
17 Helpap B: Observations on the number, size and localization of nucleoli in hyperplastic and neoplastic prostatic disease. Histopathology 1988;13:203–211.
18 Kelemen PR, Buschmann RJ, Weisz-Carrington P: Nucleolar prominence as a diagnostic variable in prostatic carcinoma. Cancer 1990; 65:1017–1020.
19 Pontes JE, Choe BK, Rose NR, Ercole C, Pierce JR Jr: Clinical evaluation of immunological methods for detection of prostatic acid phosphatase. J Urol 1981;126:363–365.
20 Lange PH, Winfield HN: Biological markers in urologic cancer. Cancer 1987;60:464–472.
21 Allhoff PE, Prope HK, Chapman CM, Lin Chi-Wey, Prout GR: Evaluation of prostate-specific acid phosphatase and prostate-specific antigen in identification of prostatic cancer. J Urol 1983;129:315–318.
22 Baak JPA: Basic points and practical aspects of the application of diagnostic morphometry. Pathol Res Pract 1984;179:193–194.

Eur Urol 1992;21(suppl 1):79–82

F. Di Silverio
G. D'Eramo
G.P. Flammia
M. Caponera
D. Macrí
A. Loreto
A. Sciarra

Department of Urology 'U. Bracci', University 'La Sapienza', Rome, Italy

# New Ultrasensitive Assay Development by Using Monoclonal Antibodies for Detecting Prostate-Specific Antigen

**Key Words**
Prostate-specific antigen
Prostate cancer
Tumor marker
Prostate cancer screening
Prostate cancer follow-up

**Abstract**
The Serono Maia Clone prostatic-specific antigen (PSA) kit incorporates an immunoradiometric assay for the measurement of PSA in the serum. The method can be used over a range of 0–100 ng/ml without dilution. Standard concentrations are 0, 0.4, 1, 5, 20, and 100 ng/ml. Up to date, 373 normal men, 89 normal women, 117 prostatic carcinoma, 98 other carcinoma, and 85 benign prostatic hypertrophy have been tested. The aim of this study is to evaluate the sensitivity and specificity of a new immunoassay method for the determination of PSA, that could be able to evaluate low levels of PSA, resulted undetectable with other methods. This ability could be useful in patients treated with hormone-suppressive therapy or after radical prostatectomy. We have collected all low values present in samples examined. With the Serono Maia Clone PSA kit only 26.7% of these have been evaluated as 'out' values as opposed to 46.5% with the Hybritech kit.

## Introduction

Investigators have searched continuously for an ideal marker for adenocarcinoma of the prostate. Application of modern immunochemistry techniques has permitted a new approach to markers to study prostatic diseases. Prostatic-specific antigen (PSA) is a protease specific to prostatic acinar cells. PSA was initially discovered in seminal plasma by Hara et al. [1] in 1971. In 1973, Li and Beling [2] were also able to isolate and purify it, in human seminal plasma, too. Wang et al. [3] isolated an antigen from prostatic tissue and demonstrated its specificity with prostate. It was identified in all prostatic tissue (normal, malignant and benign prostatic hyperplasia [BPH]) and could not be found in any other human tissue. Finally, Papsidero et al. [4] were able to identify PSA in human serum. Also, the complete gene encoding PSA has been localized to chromosome 19 [5]. Stamey et al. [6] calculated the half-life of serum PSA from data obtained in the postoperative period of radical prostatectomy. They determined the half-life to 2.2 ± 0.8 days. No found rhythmic or circadian fluctuations were found [7]. Since BPH and prostatic cancer are more prevalent in the same age range, the influence of BPH on serum PSA concentration must be considered if we want use it like a prostatic cancer marker.

All tumor markers may have diagnostic sensitivity and specificity; moreover, they do not always confirm cancer diagnosis or exclude its absence. Now there are no markers with the requirements of an ideal marker. This fact is directly correlated with the nature of the circulating marker which is not strictly related to neoplastic transformation.

Prof. Franco Di Silverio
Dipartimento di Urologia 'U. Bracci', Università degli Studi di Roma La Sapienza, Policlinico Umberto I
Viale del Policlinico, I-00161 Roma (Italy)


0302–2838/92/0215–0079
$2.75/0

The production of tumor marker and its consequent positivity in serum depend on cancer cell's characteristics and is related to the tumor mass. Also, cell differentiation, growth characteristics and associated treatments can influence marker production and secretion. PSA levels generally follow the evolution of advanced prostatic cancer; PSA shows rising levels with increasing stage in untreated prostatic cancer. However, if this marker frequently cannot add greatly to the clinician's assessment to the diagnosis of prostatic carcinoma, it can be greatly helpful in monitoring after prostatectomy or during hormonal therapy.

Presently there are different available assays for determining the serum PSA concentration. Immunoradiometric assay uses monoclonal antibodies (MAb) for separate epitopes on the PSA molecule; frequently the diluent used to prepare the standards of this kind of kit is female serum [8]. Other kits utilize a polyclonal radioimmunoassay based on the competitive protein-binding principles of Yalow and Berson [9]. This assay uses bovine albumin solution as a diluent for the standards.

The aim of this study is to evaluate the sensitivity and specificity of a new immunoassay method for the determination of PSA (Serono Maia Clone), that could be able to evaluate low levels of PSA, resulted undetectable with other methods. This ability could be particularly useful in patients treated with hormone-suppressive therapy or after radical prostatectomy. The results of the Serono Maia Clone PSA kit have been compared with those obtained with the Hybritech kit [8].

## Materials and Methods

To date, 762 serum samples have been tested. The patients examined were divided into: 89 normal women, 157 normal men under 40, 216 normal men over 40, 85 BPH, 117 prostatic cancer, and 98 other cancerous diseases. All serum samples were collected before rectal examination or other investigations that could affect PSA concentration. Also, conditions that could falsely elevate PSA values (prostatitis, acute urinary retention) have been considered.

All serum samples have been examined with both the Maia Clone and Hybritech kits. The Serono Maia Clone PSA kit incorporates an immunoradiometric assay for the measurement of PSA in the serum. The method can be used over the range 0–100 ng/ml without dilution. Standard concentrations are 0, 0.4, 1, 5, 20, and 100 ng/ml, incubation time is 2 h. Patient sample, standards and control (0.05 ml each) are reacted with a mixture of MAb to PSA (0.2 ml); one of the antibodies is labeled with $^{125}I$ while the other is attached to fluorescein.

At the end of the incubation period, separation of the immunocomplex is achieved by adding magnetic solid phase to which an antibody to fluorescein has been attached. The magnetic complex is precipitated in a magnetic field and precipitate is washed free of patient serum and of excess antibodies. The residual precipitate is measured using an automated gamma counter. Concentration of PSA measured is directly proportional to the radioactivity bound by separation.

Human PSA was from Scantibodies Lab. Inc. (Santee, Calif., USA); FITC (Isomer I) was from Sigma (St. Louis, Mo., USA); Protein A-Sepharose CL4B was from Pharmacia (Uppsala, Sweden), and Na-$^{125}I$ was from New England Nuclear (Boston, Mass., USA).

*PSA standard:* Pooled, filtered to 0.22 µm, 1 g/l sodium azide added; bovine serum was from Miles.

*PSA wash buffer:* The wash buffer was sodium phosphate (2 mmol/l, pH 7.0) containing per liter, 5 g bovine serum albumin, Cohn fraction V, 150 mmol sodium chloride, and 2 mmol sodium azide.

*Monoclonal antibodies:* Two MAb present in the kit tracer were both IgG1 isotypes; they were purified by protein A-Sepharose CL4B and eluted in Na citrate 0.1 *M* at pH 5.5, then dialyzed in PBS, pH 7.2.

*Preparation of $^{125}I$-labeled antibodies:* MAb were labeled by the lactoperoxidase procedure to contain an average of 0.8 atoms of $^{125}I$ per antibody molecule. The reaction was blocked by 2 mg of $NaN_3$. Protein separation from unreacted iodine was achieved by gel filtration on Superose 12, FPLC.

*Preparation of FITC-labeled antibodies:* FITC and MAb were mixed in sodium bicarbonate, 0.2 *M,* pH 9.0, in a ratio of 1:20 FITC vs. MAb, respectively. Protein separation from unreacted FITC was achieved by desalting in a column containing Sephadex G-25, 26 × 100 cm, being eluted at 90 ml/l. FITC-conjugated antibody, which eluted in the void volume, incorporated approximately seven molecules of FITC per IgG molecule. Anti-FITC solid phase was purchased from Serono Diagnostic SA (Coinsins, Switzerland), and was used at a concentration of antiserum anti-FITC raised in sheep.

## Results

*Distribution Observed in Normal Women.* Utilizing the Serono Maia Clone kit (MS), in 83.1% of cases we found undetectable PSA values; utilizing the Hybritech kit (HY) we also found undetectable values, namely 85.4%. Utilizing the MS kit there were no patients with a PSA value over 1 ng/ml and only 1.1% with the HY kit (table 1).

*Distribution Observed in Normal Men Under and Over 40.* In normal men under 40, 95.7% of cases with MS against 87.1% with HY has shown a PSA value between 0 and 1 ng/ml (table 2). In normal men over 40, PSA values between 0 and 1 ng/ml have been found in 82% and 68.7% of cases, respectively, utilizing the MS and HY kits. Only 3.7% presented values over 3 ng/ml (table 3).

*Distribution Observed in BPH Patients.* Measurement in BPH patients has shown that in 69.2% with MS against 68.4% with HY, PSA values were between 0 and 3 ng/ml. Only 6% (MS) and 6.8% (HY) respectively presented values over 10 ng/ml (table 4).

**Table 1.** Distribution of PSA values observed in normal women

| | | |
|---|---|---|
| MS | 83.1% | 0% |
| HY | 85.4% | 1.1% |
| PSA | 0 ng/ml | > 1 ng/ml |

**Table 2.** Distribution of PSA values observed in normal men under 40

| | | |
|---|---|---|
| MS | 95.7% | 4.28% |
| HY | 87.1% | 12.8% |
| PSA | 0–1 ng/ml | 1–3 ng/ml |

**Table 3.** Distribution of PSA values observed in normal men over 40

| | | | |
|---|---|---|---|
| MS | 82% | 13.7% | 3.7% |
| HY | 68.7% | 27.5% | 3.7% |
| PSA | 0–1 ng/ml | 1–3 ng/ml | > 3 ng/ml |

**Table 4.** Distribution of PSA values observed in BPH patients

| | | | |
|---|---|---|---|
| MS | 69.2% | 24.8% | 6% |
| HY | 68.4% | 24.8% | 6.8% |
| PSA | 0–3 ng/ml | 3–10 ng/ml | > 10 ng/ml |

**Table 5.** Distribution of PSA values observed in nonprostatic cancer patients

| | | | |
|---|---|---|---|
| MS | 89.8% | 9.2% | 1% |
| HY | 86.7% | 12.2% | 1% |
| PSA | 0–3 ng/ml | 3–10 ng/ml | > 10 ng/ml |

**Table 6.** Distribution of PSA values observed in prostatic cancer

| | | | |
|---|---|---|---|
| MS | 54.1% | 21.2% | 24.7% |
| HY | 51.8% | 22.3% | 25.9% |
| PSA | 0–3 ng/ml | 3–10 ng/ml | > 10 ng/ml |

*Distribution Observed in Nonprostatic Cancer Patients.* 89.8% (MS) against 86.7% (HY) of patients has shown values between 0 and 3 ng/ml. PSA values were over 10 ng/ml in only 1% (table 5).

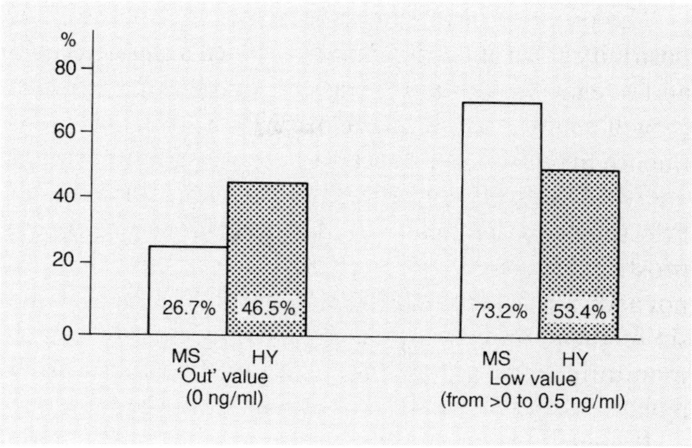


**Fig. 1.** Distribution observed in low PSA values (range 0–0.5 ng/ml).

*Distribution Observed in Prostatic Cancer.* In 54.1% (MS) against 51.8% (HY) of all prostatic cancer cases, we have found PSA values between 0 and 3 ng/ml; 24.7% (MS) against 25.9% (HY) was over 10 ng/ml (table 6). To determine the sensitivity of this new immunoassay method (Serono Maia Clone), we have collected all low values (range 0–0.5 ng/ml) present in the samples examined and have verified its ability to evaluate this range. With the Serono Maia Clone PSA kit, only 26.7% of these cases has been evaluated as having an 'Out' value, against 46.5% with the Hybritech kit. Moreover, in 73% with MS against 53.4% with HY, we have found dosable values from > 0 to 0.5 ng/ml (fig. 1).

## Conclusion

The Serono Maia Clone PSA kit has been able to evaluate lower PSA levels than the Hybritech PSA kit, either in control patients or in patients with BPH or prostatic cancer [10]. This result is especially significant in the evaluation of prostatic cancer after radical prostatectomy or during hormonal therapy. In fact, the nadir of PSA is of considerable prognostic importance; the patients whose PSA fell to normal levels, or better to undetectable levels, have the best chance of a prolonged response to treatment. This immunoassay method can increase the clinical usefulness of PSA in monitoring patients after definitive therapy. With prostatectomy, if all prostatic tissue is removed, the serum concentration of PSA should decrease to zero or become undetectable. Depending upon the assay used, the definition of a positive PSA value (serum level indicative of residual disease) after radical prostatectomy can vary. It is very important then to determine an appropriate cut-off level. This level normally ranges from 0.2 to 0.6 ng/ml [11–14].

The Serono Maia Clone PSA kit was able to evaluate 42.5% of samples as being 'Out' for the Hybritech PSA kit, increasing the possibility to identify the presence of residual disease.

In the Johns Hopkins' experience, all patients with a documented local recurrence or distant metastasis had an elevated postoperative PSA level; on the contrary, no patient with undetectable PSA concentration had evidence of recurrent disease [15]. Kuriyama et al. [16] demonstrated that PSA may be clinically useful to predict prognosis and monitoring to hormonal treatment in patients with prostatic cancer. In these patients, PSA concentrations are inversely related to survival time. Moreover, during the treatment, PSA levels increase when the cancer progresses and decreases during remission periods. In fact, the positive response to hormonal therapy produces a precipitous decrease in the serum PSA concentration.

Ercole et al. [17] reported a decrease in PSA levels of stage D2 prostatic cancer from 85 to 2.1 ng/ml. Instead, 88% of clinically active stage D2 after endocrine therapy had PSA values over 10 ng/ml [18]. Also, bone scintigraphy is an important criterion in the assessment of response in advanced disease [19]. Hetherington et al. [20] examined the relationship between PSA values and bone scintigraphy in 120 patients. Of 54 with negative bone scans, 10 developed skeletal metastases and PSA were rising in 9 of these patients. In 66 cases with documented metastases, bone scan evidence of progression was seen in 36 and PSA was rising in 72% of cases.

The correct use of markers can improve our ability to have a prognostic indicator to prostatic cancer. This kit has shown a high sensitivity and specificity for the determination of PSA levels, that could be particularly capable of distinguishing patients with a favorable and persisting response to androgen blockade therapy, or predicting new progression in patients with partial response.


## Acknowledgements

We would like to recognize the contribution of Drs G. Fiorani and A. Nastari (Serono Industries) for their precious technical support.


## References


1 Hara M, Inorre T, Fukuyama T: Some physicochemical characteristics of gamma-seminoprotein, an antigen component specific for human seminal plasma. Jpn J Leg Med 1971;25:322.

2 Li TS, Beling CG: Isolation and characterization of two specific antigens of human seminal plasma. Fertil Steril 1973;24:134.

3 Wang MC, Valenzuela LA, Murphy GP, Chu TM: Purification of a human prostate-specific antigen. Invest Urol 1979;17:159.

4 Papsidero LD, Wang MC, Valenzuela MA, Murphy GP, Chu TM: A prostate antigen in sera of prostatic cancer patients. Cancer Res 1980;40:2428.

5 Riegman PHJ, Vliestra RJ, van der Korpert JA, Romijn JC, Trapman J: Characterization of the prostate-specific antigen gene: a novel human kallikrein-like gene. Biochem Biophys Res Commun 1989;159:95.

6 Stamey TA, Yang N, Hay AR, McNeal JE, Freiha FS, Redwine E: Prostate-specific antigen as a serum marker for adenocarcinoma of the prostate. N Engl J Med 1987;317:909.

7 Lindstedt G, Jacobsson A, Lundberg PA, Hedelin H, Pettersson S, Unsgaard B: Determination of prostate-specific antigen in serum by immunoradiometric assay. Clin Chem 1990; 36:53.

8 Myrtle JF, Klimley PG, Ivor LP, Brun JF: Clinical utility of prostate-specific antigen in the management of prostate cancer. Adv Cancer Diag. Hybritech Inc, 1986.

9 Yalow RS, Berson SA: Introduction and general considerations; in Odell WD (ed): Principles of Competitive Protein Binding Assays. Philadelphia, Lippincott, 1971, chapt 1, pp 1–24.

10 Di Silverio F, D'Eramo G, Flammia GP, Sciarra A, Macrí D, Caponera M: New ultrasensitive assay development by using monoclonal antibodies for detecting PSA. Eur Urol 1991;19(suppl):2.

11 Stamey TA, Kabalin JN, McNeal JE, Johnstone IM, Freiha F, Redwine EA, Yang N: Prostate-specific antigen in the diagnosis and treatment of adenocarcinoma of the prostate. Radical prostatectomy-treated patients. J Urol 1989;141:1076.

12 Hudson MA, Bahnson RR, Catalona WJ: Clinical use of prostate-specific antigen in patients with prostate cancer. J Urol 1989;142:1011.

13 Lange PH, Ercole CJ, Lightner DJ, Fraley EE, Vessella R: The value of serum prostate-specific antigen determinations before and after radical prostatectomy. J Urol 1989;141:873.

14 Carter HB, Partin AW, Oesterling JE, Weber JP, Epstein JI, Chan DW, Rock RC, Walsh PC: The use of prostate-specific antigen in the management of patients with prostate cancer. The Johns Hopkins' experience; in Catalona WJ (ed): Clinical Aspects of Prostate Cancer. New York, 1989, pp 247–254.

15 Morgan WR, Zincke H, Rainwater LM, Myers RP, Klee GG: Prostate-specific antigen values after radical retropubic prostatectomy for adenocarcinoma of the prostate: impact of adjuvant treatment (hormonal and radiation). J Urol 1991;145:319.

16 Kuriyama M, Wang MC, Lee CL, Killian CS, Papsidero LD, Inaji H, Loor RM, Lin MF, Nishiura T, Slack NH, Murphy GP, Chu TM: Use of human prostate-specific antigen in monitoring prostate cancer. Cancer Res 1981; 41:3874.

17 Ercole CJ, Lange PH, Mathisen M, Chiou RK, Reddy PK, Vessella RL: Prostate-specific antigen and prostatic acid phosphatase in the monitoring and staging of patients with prostatic cancer. J Urol 1987;138:1181.

18 Weber JP, Oesterlin JE, Peters CA, Partin AW, Chan DW, Walsh PC: The influence of reversible androgen deprivation on serum prostate-specific antigen levels in men with benign prostatic hyperplasia. J Urol 1989;141:987.

19 Cooper EH, Armitage TG: Tumour markers in monitoring the treatment of advanced prostate cancer; in Schroeder FH (ed): Treatment of Prostatic Cancer: Facts and Controversies. EORTC Monogr 8. Prog Clin Biol Res 1989; 359.

20 Hetherington JW, Siddall JK, Cooper EH: Contribution of bone scintigraphy and prostate-specific antigen to the monitoring of prostatic cancer. Eur Urol 1988;14:1–5.

Eur Urol 1992;21(suppl 1):83–86

*I. Romics*
*L. Galamb*

Department of Urology,
Semmelweis Medical University,
Budapest, Hungary, and Municipal
Hospital, Fulda, FRG

# Changes in Prostate-Specific Antigen and Prostatic Acid Phosphatase Concentration following Prostatic Examination in Benign Prostatic Hypertrophy and Prostate Cancer Patients

**Key Words**
Prostate-specific antigen
Prostatic acid phosphatase
Benign prostatic hypertrophy
Prostate cancer
Rectal digital investigation
Cystoscopy
Punch biopsy

**Abstract**
The authors measured serum prostate-specific antigen (PSA) and prostatic acid phosphatase concentration in histologically positive prostate hyperplastic and carcinomatous patients before, and 30–60 min and 24 h after prostate manipulation (rectal digital examination, cystoscopy and perineal punch biopsy). After rectal examination, PSA, and after other interventions, both markers changed significantly, although in different points of time and to a different extent. The authors call the attention to the importance of the point of time of the examination. Examination following prostate manipulation may result in wrong diagnosis or in erroneous therapeutic consequences in the follow-up period.

The significance of prostate-specific antigen (PSA) and of prostatic acid phosphatase (PAP) determined with immunological methods in the diagnosis of prostate cancer and in the follow-up period was described by several authors [3, 4, 6] and our results coincide with the international results [9]. Experience of potential errors of the investigation is very important as erroneously high values of benign prostatic hypertrophy (BPH) patients refer to malignancy, or give incorrect information on progression or regression trends in the follow-up period. This may involve serious therapeutic consequences. So we deemed it important to investigate how the PSA and PAP concentrations are changing in the serum of BPH and prostate carcinoma (PCA) patients after prostatic manipulation.

## Material and Methods

Histologically proven 35 BPH and 29 PCA patients were investigated. Changes in the marker concentration were caused by three different interventions – rectal digital examination, cystoscopy and perineal punch biopsy were studied. As not all the three examinations were performed in all patients, the data are demonstrated in table 1. PAP and PSA values were measured 48 h prior to, and 30–60 min and 24 h after the examination. Measurements were performed with the help of Tandem PAP and Tandem PSA kits (Hybritech, USA). The upper limit of the normal values is beyond 2.0 μg/ml in the case of PAP and beyond 4.0 μg/ml in the case of PSA. Two measurements were made from each sample and an average value was calculated. Statistical evaluation was made with the help of the 'simple F comparisons' method.

I. Romics, MD, PhD
Department of Urology
Semmelweis Medical University
Üllői-út 78/b, H–1082 Budapest (Hungary)


0302–2838/92/0215–0083
$2.75/0

**Table 1.** Investigations performed in our patients

| | PSA | PAP |
|---|---|---|
| *BPH* | | |
| Rectal digital | 14 | 17 |
| Cystoscopy | 9 | 10 |
| Perineal biopsy | 7 | 8 |
| *PCA* | | |
| Rectal digital | 10 | 10 |
| Cystoscopy | 7 | 7 |
| Perineal biopsy | 12 | 12 |

**Table 2.** Results

| | Prostate hyperplasy | Prostate carcinoma |
|---|---|---|
| Rectal examination | | |
| PAP | not significant | not significant |
| PSA | p0 vs. o24 = p < 0.05 | p0 vs. p30 = p < 0.001<br>p0 30 vs. o24 = p < 0.05 |
| Cystoscopy | | |
| PAP | p0 vs. p30 = p < 0.05<br>p0 vs. p60 = p < 0.05<br>p0 vs. o24 = p < 0.01 | not significant |
| PSA | p0 vs. p30 = p < 0.01<br>p0 vs. p60 = p < 0.001<br>p0 vs. o24 = p < 0.01 | p0 vs. p60 = p < 0.01 |
| PAP | p0 vs. p30 = p < 0.05 | p0 vs. p60 = p < 0.05<br>p0 vs. o24 = p < 0.02 |
| PSA | p0 vs. p60 = p < 0.01<br>p30 vs. p60 = p < 0.01<br>p30 vs. o24 = p < 0.02 | p0 vs. p30 = p < 0.0001<br>p0 vs. p60 = p < 0.0001<br>p0 vs. o24 = p < 0.0001<br>p30 vs. o24 = p < 0.0001<br>p60 vs. o24 = p < 0.003 |

p0 = Prior to examination; p30 = 30 min following examination; p60 = 60 min following examination; o24 = 24 h following examination.

## Results

Figures 1 and 2 demonstrate the marker changes caused by rectal digital examination in BPH and PCA patients. PAP did not change in either of the groups. Maximum PSA concentration values in BPH patients were measured after 24 h. In PCA patients, maximum concentration was to be observed 30 min after the rectal manipulation. The changes were significant. Considerable PAP and PSA changes were observed both 30–60 min and 24 h after cystoscopy in BPH patients. Maximum PSA concentration was measured 1 h after the rectal manipulation; PAP could be measured 24 h after cystoscopy. In case of PCA, only the PSA increase was significant after 60 min. It should be taken into account that the scattering is far greater in the case of PCA patients (fig. 3, 4). Perineal biopsy increased PAP concentration in BHP patients in the 30th minute. PSA concentration reached its maximum value in the 60th minute and a similarly high concentration was to be measured even after 24 h. Changes in the PAP value were more prominent in PCA patients. PSA increased abruptly after biopsy and increased continuously up to the 24th hour. Statistical examination shows very high significance (fig. 5, 6). Marker results and the results of statistical examinations are summarized in table 2.

## Discussion

PSA and PAP determined by immunological methods became the most important markers of prostatic patients and routine examinations of urology [5]. The changes in the concentration of prostate-specific tumor markers are influenced by different factors.

Marker concentrations before and after radical prostatectomy were measured by Lange et al. [7]. Connection between the grading of the tumor and the marker was stated by Haapainen et al. [2], while between the size of the tumor and the marker concentration by Stamey et al. [11]. The above relates to PCA patients, but the markers were also studied in BPH and in prostatic patients [10].

Vesey et al. [12] investigated PAP and PSA concentrations in PCA patients after transurethral resection of the prostate (TUR). Significant concentration increase was to be measured in BPH patients, but the same could not be observed in PCA patients after TUR. Marker concentrations are also influenced by drug and X-ray treatment. We ourselve examined the PSA and PAP concentration changes following rather certain routine examinations than different therapeutic methods. Rectal palpation did not show changes in PAP.

In more than 50% of the cases of El-Shirbiny et al. [1] PAP concentration increased after palpation. They did not make a statistical analysis and in the lack of such analysis the extent of changes cannot be evaluated.

Pearson [8] and Wadström et al. [13] observed a significant PAP increase after prostate massage. Stamey et al.

1
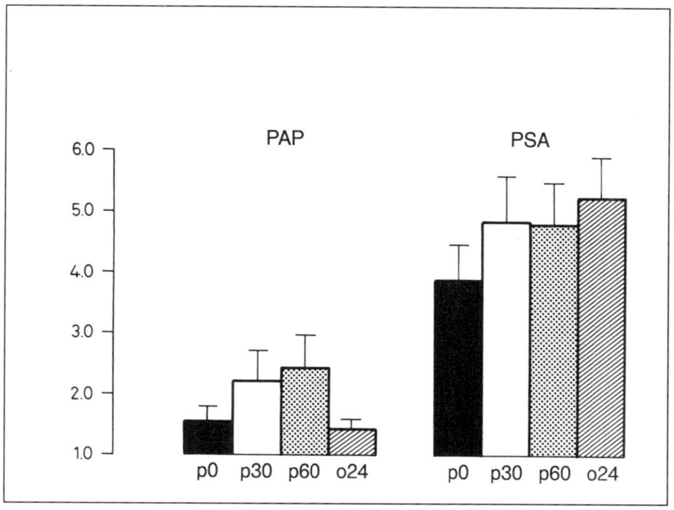


2
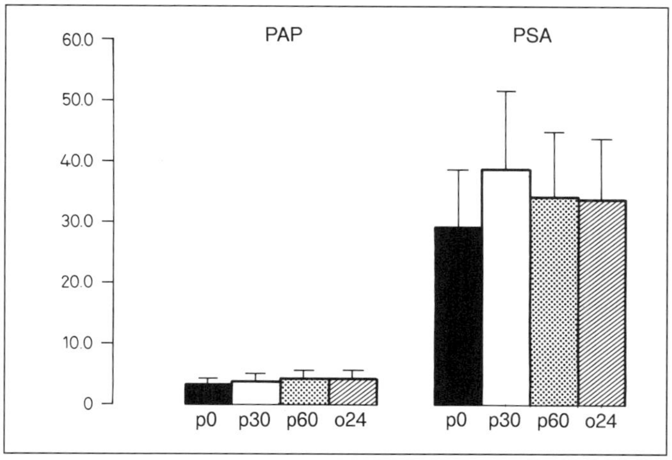


3
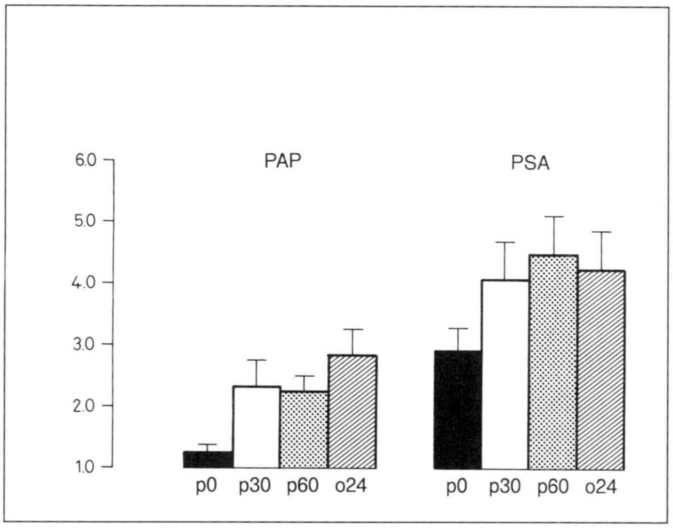


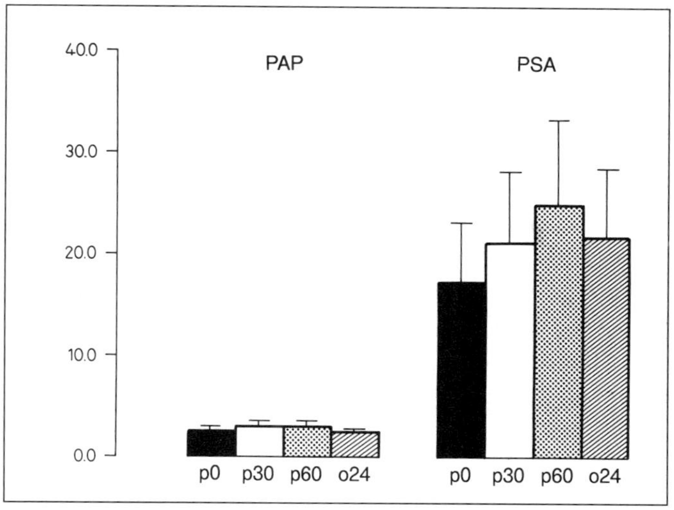

4

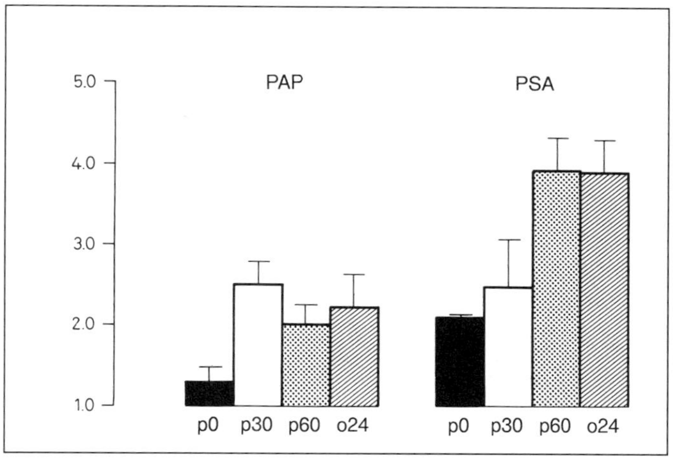

5

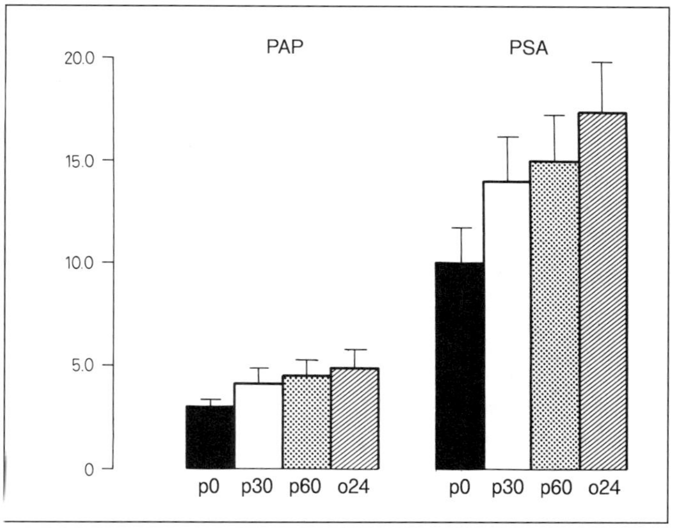

6

**Fig. 1.** Changes in PSA and PAP concentration in BPH patients following rectal palpitation.

**Fig. 2.** Changes in tumor markers in PCA patients following rectal examination.

**Fig. 3.** Changes in markers due to cystoscopy in BPH patients.

**Fig. 4.** Changes in markers following cystocopy of PCA patients.

**Fig. 5.** Changes in markers following perineal prostate biopsy in BPH patients.

**Fig. 6.** Results of marker measurements prior to and after perineal biopsy in PCA patients.

[11] reported on a significant PSA concentration increase following massage. In our material the significant concentration increase in BPH patients after 24 h points out to the fact that blood sampling for PSA the day after the admission, i.e. after the clinical examination, so among others palpation, is too early and that one should wait at least 2 days before blood sampling. In PCA patients we will get higher starting values if PSA examination takes place 24 h after palpitation. This does not cause any problem in the follow-up period.

Cystoscopy certainly exerts a greater physical effect than palpation. Both markers showed significant changes in BPH patients. In PCA patients, PAP did not change significantly and even PSA changed only in one point of time, i.e. in the 60th minute. No doubt, the essence of BPH is obstruction and the instrument must be forced through the pars prostatica narrowed down by the lateral and intermediate lobes. PCA does not always involve obstruction; maybe this is an explanation – however rather speculative – for the results obtained. Anyway, we would like to call again the attention on the possibility and risk of erroneous measurement in BPH patients.

The following conclusions can be drawn from the results: Rectal digital examination does not change PAP concentration either in BPH or in PCA patients. PSA increases to a slightly significant extent in BPH patients. The main point is that while the values prior to examination were beyond the normal upper limit, the average values after prostate palpation reached the pathologic rate.

Average PSA values in BPH patients were higher than the normal after cystoscopy as well. After cystoscopy all the measuring results reached the domain of tumor, but due to the relatively low number of cases and to the wide scattering, significant change was experienced only in one point of time.

Biopsy exerts less influence on PAP concentration than on the quantitative change of PSA in the serum. In the majority of casses we observed significant PSA increase 24 h following the examination. Consequently, we can state that the measuring of tumor markers within 48 h following the instrumental or manual prostate examination is not advisable. Even we ourselves did not believe that it would be expedient to repeat the measurements after 48 h and in later points of time. Further investigations are needed to recognize and eliminate errors arising in the course of clinical and laboratory works.

## References


1 El-Shirbiny AM, Shridhar P, Al Adnani MS, Shures LK: Enzyme immunoassay of prostatic acid phosphatase after prostatic examination. Urology 1988;32:469.

2 Haapainen RK, Permi EJ, Ranniko SAS, Voutilainen PEJ, Alfthan OS: Prostate tumour markers and differentiation grade in prostatic cancer. Br J Urol 1990;66:635.

3 Huber PR, Hering F, Rist M, Misteli R, Rutishauser G: Prostate-specific antigen: Experimental and clinical data. Urol Res 1986;14:164.

4 Killian CS, Emrich LJ, Vargas FP, Kuriyama M, Wang MC, Slack NH, Papsidero LD, Murphy GP, Chu TM: Prognostic importance of prostate-specific antigen for monitoring patients with stage B2 to D1 prostate cancer. Cancer Res 1985;45:886.

5 Knönagel H, Gautsch K, Vonderschmitt DJ, Hauri D: Der Wert des prostataspezifischen Antigens im Vergleich zur sauren Prostataphosphatase in der Diagnose des Prostatakarzinoms. Aktuel Urol 1988;19:89.

6 Kuriyyama M, Wang MC, Lee CL, Papsidero LP, Killian CS: Use of human prostate-specific antigen in monitoring prostate cancer. Cancer Res 1981;41:3874.

7 Lange H, Ercole CJ, Lightner DJ, Fraley EE, Vessella R: The value of serum prostate-specific antigen determination before and after radical prostatectomy. J Urol 1989;141:873.

8 Pearson IJ: Radioimmunoassay of serum prostatic acid phosphatase after prostatic massage. Urology 1983;21:37.

9 Romics I, Bach D: Experience with prostate-specific antigen in prostatic carcinoma. Int Urol Nephrol 1991;23:465.

10 Seamonds B, Yang N, Anderson K, Whitaker B, Shaw LA, Bollinger JR: Evaluation of prostatic-specific antigen and prostatic acid phosphatase as prostate cancer markers. Urology 1986;28:472.

11 Stamey TA, Yang N, Hay AR, McNeal JE, Freiha LK: Prostate-specific antigen as a serum marker for adenocarcinoma of the prostate. N Engl J Med 1987;317:909.

12 Vesey SG, Goble NM, Stower MJ, Hammonds JC, Smith PJB: The effect of transurethral prostatectomy on serum prostate-specific antigen. Br J Urol 1988;62:347.

13 Wadström H, Huber P, Rutishauser G: Elevation of serum prostatic acid phosphatase after prostatic massage. Urology 1984;24:550.

Eur Urol 1992;21(suppl 1):87–91

*Paolo Puppo*[a]
*Massimo Perachino*[a]
*Giuseppe Ricciotti*[a]
*Alessandro Vitali*[b]
*Silvia Arduino*[b]
*Lucia Di Ciolo*[c]

Departments of
[a] Urology,
[b] Pathology and
[c] Nuclear Medicine, S. Corona Hospital,
Pietra Ligure (SV), Italy

# Comparison between Digital Rectal Examination, Prostate-Specific Antigen and Transrectal Ultrasound in Symptomatic Patients

**Results on 141 Cases**

**Key Words**
Prostate cancer
Transrectal ultrasound
Prostate-specific antigen

**Abstract**
In this study we proposed to verify sensitivity and specificity of prostate-specific antigen (PSA), digital rectal examination (DRE) and transrectal ultrasound (TRUS) in patients who referred at our institution for prostatic complaints. 141 patients, ages ranging between 55 and 86 years (mean 67.5), underwent DRE, blood PSA, TRUS and ultrasonically guided biopsy of the prostate. The comparison of the results obtained with the different diagnostic tools allowed us to draw a diagnostic algorithm for prostate cancer in symptomatic patients.

## Introduction

Since the death rate for prostate cancer continues to increase [1], new methods for early detection should be evaluated. In 1980, Guinan et al. [2] compared digital rectal examination (DRE) to other diagnostic tests and concluded that it was the most accurate. In 1988, Lee et al. [3] showed transrectal ultrasound (TRUS) to be twice as sensitive for prostate cancer detection as DRE. Prostate-specific antigen (PSA), a glycoprotein, is considered a sensitive marker for prostate cancer and has been proposed for monitoring the response of prostate cancer to therapy, while its role in diagnosis is yet to be defined.

## Materials and Methods

Between September 1990 and June 1991, 141 patients with prostatic symptoms underwent PSA determination, DRE and TRUS. Ages ranged between 55 and 86 years (mean 67.5). All TRUS has been performed in sagittal and longitudinal projections with a Brüel & Kjaer Model 1846 scanner with use of a 7.5-MHz multiplane probe.

Ultrasonically guided biopsies have been done via the transrectal route using an automatic biopsy system (Biopsy-Cut, needle 18 gauge, 20 cm; Bard Urological Division).

In all cases, we performed the following procedures in this order: (1) Before any manipulation of the prostate, a blood sample was obtained for PSA determination with the Hybritech technique (normal values $< 3.5$ ng/ml). (2) DRE is obtained and recorded on the day of TRUS examination. (3) TRUS: if TRUS was considered suspicious, the ultrasonographic stage of the hypoechoic lesion was registered according to Lee et al. [6]: UA $< 1$ cm, UB1 1–1.5 cm, UB2 $> 1.5$ cm.

Dr. Paolo Puppo
Department of Urology
S. Corona Hospital
I-17027 Pietra Ligure/sv (Italy)


0302–2838/92/0215–0087
$2.75/0

**Table 1.** Sensitivity and specificity of different diagnostic tools (n = 141)

| | Sensitivity | Specificity |
|---|---|---|
| PSA | 72.9% | 62.3% |
| DRE | 68.7% | 44.1% |
| TRUS | 91.6% | 54.3% |

All evaluated patients underwent ultrasonically guided biopsy, with a mean of 2.7 scores (max. 6, min. 1) obtained. Therefore, we could calculate sensitivity and specificity of DRE, PSA and TRUS in our series.

*Statistical Analysis.* The histological results of biopsies constitute the standard of comparison for the calculation of sensitivity and specificity of different tests. Sensitivity was defined as the percentage of positive tests in patients with proven prostate cancer. Specificity was defined as the percentage of negative tests in patients with negative biopsies.

## Results

All 141 biopsies were performed via the transrectal route, with no major complications; mild fever (<38.5 °C) was observed in 16 cases (11.3%), and resolved in a few days with common antibiotics. In 7 cases (4.9%) there was macroscopic self-limited hematuria, lasting for no more than 3 days.

Chemoprophylaxis with 2 g piperacillin i.m., once only 1 h before the biopsy, was used in 89 cases (63.1%), while in the remaining cases no prophylaxis was used without complications. In 48 cases (34.5%) biopsy revealed a prostate cancer, and in the remaining 93 cases (65.5%) benign prostatic hypertrophy or prostatitis was found. We excluded from statistical analysis the cases that revealed dysplasia or prostatic intraepithelial neoplasia (PIN). Results are presented separately for every diagnostic tool and then in comparison.

### *TRUS Alone*

TRUS was considered positive in 87 cases of 141 patients (61.7%). Criterion of positivity was hypoechoic lesion visualized in both longitudinal and transverse planes. In case of considered negative TRUS, at least 5 random biopsies were taken. In 44 of 48 cases of proven prostate cancer, TRUS was considered positive (sensitivity of 91.6%); 50 out of 93 cases of negative biopsies were associated with negative TRUS (specificity of 54.3%) (table 1).

### *PSA Alone*

PSA was positive (> 3.5 ng/ml) in 71 out of 141 cases (50.3%). PSA was > 10 ng/ml in 25 cases (17.7%); in 24 cases it was associated with cancer (96%) at biopsy, and all with positive TRUS. PSA sensitivity was 72.9% (35 cases out of 48), and its specificity was 62.3% (58 cases out of 93) (table 1).

### *DRE Alone*

The DRE, in our series, was considered suspicious in 84 of 141 cases (59.6%). DRE sensitivity was 68.7% (33 cases out of 48), and specificity was 44.1% (41 cases out of 93) (table 1).

*DRE–PSA–.* In 25 cases (17.7%), PSA and DRE were both negative. In 12 cases (48%) TRUS was considered positive. One patient (4%) had a prostate cancer: TRUS was negative in this case. Therefore, in this group of patients there was a 4% chance of tumor irrespective of TRUS (tables 2, 3).

*DRE+PSA–.* In 45 cases (31.9%), DRE was suspicious and PSA was negative. In 28 cases (62.2%) TRUS was considered positive. In these patients, 9 tumors were found at biopsy (20%): 1 out of 9 tumors was associated with negative TRUS (2.2%). In these patients the cumulative chance of harboring a tumor was 20%; if TRUS was negative, we had 5.9% of tumors (1 case out of 17). In case of positive TRUS, the tumor percentage increases to 28.6% (8 cases out of 28) (tables 2, 3).

*PSA+DRE–.* In 32 cases (22.7%), PSA was positive and associated with negative DRE. Biopsies revealed 10 tumors (31.2%): in 2 tumors TRUS was negative (6.2%), but PSA was > 10 ng/ml. Given a cumulative tumor rate of 31.2%, the tumor percentage falls to 12.5% (2/16) if TRUS was negative and increases to 50% with positive TRUS (8/16) (tables 2, 3).

*PSA+DRE+.* In 39 cases (27.6%), PSA and DRE were both positive. TRUS was positive in 31 cases (79.4%). 28 biopsies were positive (71.8%); 100% of tumors were associated with positive TRUS. In these patients, in case of negative TRUS there was a 25% chance of finding a tumor (2/8), while with positive TRUS the percentage was 83.9 (26/31) (tables 2, 3).

**Table 2.** Number of tumors found at biopsy and tumor rates of different results of DRE and PSA with regard to TRUS (n = 141)

| | DRE–PSA– (n = 25) | | DRE–PSA+ (n = 32) | | DRE+SPA– (n = 45) | | DRE+PSA+ (n = 39) | |
|---|---|---|---|---|---|---|---|---|
| | n | % | n | % | n | % | n | % |
| TRUS– | 1/13 | 7.6 | 2/16 | 12.5 | 1/17 | 5.9 | 2/8 | 25.0 |
| TRUS+ | 0/12 | 0 | 8/16 | 50.0 | 8/28 | 28.6 | 26/31 | 83.9 |

**Table 3.** Number of tumors found at biopsy and cumulative tumor rates irrespective of TRUS compared to the different results of DRE and PSA

| | DRE–PSA– (n = 25) | | DRE–PSA+ (n = 32) | | DRE+PSA– (n = 45) | | DRE+PSA+ (n = 39) | |
|---|---|---|---|---|---|---|---|---|
| | n | % | n | % | n | % | n | % |
| Tumors at biopsy | 1/15 | 4.0 | 10/32 | 31.2 | 9/45 | 20.0 | 28/39 | 71.7 |

## Discussion

The continued upward trend of mortality for prostate cancer emphasizes the need to detect it at an earlier stage [1]. As for other tumors, we should need an ideal serum tumor marker, that is one expressed only by cancer cells and that can be detected with reliability at the time the tumor achieves biological importance [9, 10, 12].

However, this perfect tumor marker has not yet been discovered. As it has been discussed already, PSA is not prostate cancer-specific; it is prostate tissue-specific and as a result numerous benign conditions of the prostate can influence its serum concentration [12, 13]. In addition, numerous studies suggested that not all prostate cancers cause a detectable elevation in the serum PSA level [10, 11, 14, 15].

Thus, the usefulness of PSA, by itself, in the detection of curable prostate cancers may be limited [4–7, 16]. In fact, we found a fairly good sensitivity of PSA alone (72.9%), in contrast with a poor specificity (62.3%); when considering only the cases in which PSA was more than 10 ng/ml, we had a 96% chance of finding a prostate cancer at biopsy (24 cases out of 25); we must consider that this group of patients has generally high stage tumors, with also suspicious DRE or positive TRUS.

Our findings are similar to those reported in the literature. Cooner et al. [18], using the same Hybritech assay, reported a PSA sensitivity and specificity of 75% and 79.7%, respectively. Using the same technique, Hudson et al. [14] reported a 70% sensitivity and a 77% specificity.

In our setting, TRUS alone showed a better sensitivity than PSA alone (91.6%), with a lower specificity (54.3%). Our figures are similar to those obtained by Cooner et al. [18] in a screening setting on 225 patients; they had a TRUS sensitivity and specificity of 100% and 65%, respectively; Devonec et al. [19], in a clinical setting on 213 patients, found a 48% sensitivity and a 65% specificity for TRUS.

DRE in our hands showed a sensitivity of 68.7% and a specificity of 44.1%. Lee et al. [3] on a screening study found a 45.5% sensitivity and a 97.5% specificity for DRE on 784 men; these figures are different from ours, probably because the values of sensitivity and specificity have been obtained by calculating the estimated prevalence of prostate cancer in a healthy population and assuming that all tumors of a finite size in that cohort of men were found with use of both TRUS and DRE.

In fact, as pointed out by Cooner [17], we must take care to understand the difference between screening and cancer detection in patients who are under the care of a physician. While the efficacy of the screening test is yet to be determined, the detection of cancer among patients in whom the physician is assessing clinical information, physical examination, serum markers, and TRUS is quite another matter.

Whenever the slightest suspicion of prostate cancer exists, ultrasonically guided transrectal needle biopsy affords a simple, painless, accurate and relatively innocuous method of determining its significance. Anyway, combining DRE with the results of TRUS and PSA values, we can detect more early, curable prostate cancers [7, 8]. In

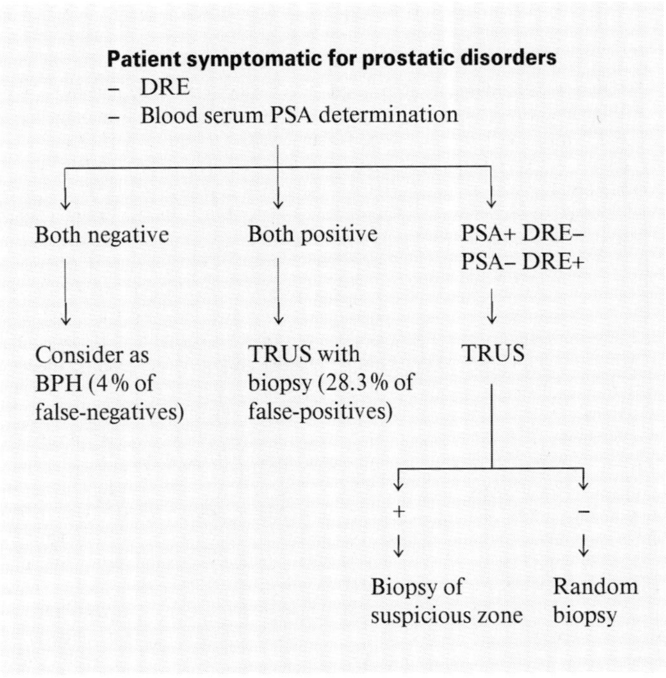


**Fig. 1.** Prostate cancer detection algorithm in symptomatic patients.

our setting, a normal PSA coupled with a normal DRE (25 patients) gave a tumor detection rate of 4% (1 case); in this case TRUS had been considered negative. In such patients TRUS seems questionable for cancer detection purposes and however, biopsy should be taken only in patients with positive TRUS.

A normal PSA coupled with a suspicious DRE yielded a detection rate of 20% (9 tumors out of 45 patients). Eight tumors were associated with suspicious TRUS, while only 1 tumor was associated with negative TRUS (1 out of 17, 5.9%). In this group of patients it should seem mandatory to perform an ultrasonically guided biopsy in case of suspicious TRUS; in case of negative TRUS, it seems to be questionable to perform a biopsy on the suspicious palpable nodule. However, Lee et al. [3] found 15% of palpable tumors with negative TRUS in a screening study.

A 6% chance of finding a cancer in DRE+PSA–TRUS– patients suggests to perform a biopsy of the palpable nodule; in fact, if the biopsy reveals positive, the cancer is almost certainly within the gland and potentially curable. PSA elevation to any degree produced a cumulative detection rate of 31.2% in DRE– patients, and one of 71.8% in DRE+ patients. In patients with PSA+ and DRE–, if TRUS was negative the tumor rate was 12.5%; the value increased to 50% if TRUS was suspicious.

Cooner et al. [7] found a 35% of cancer detection in patients with abnormal PSA and suspicious TRUS and a 19.6% of cancer in cases with abnormal PSA and normal TRUS. Therefore, in these patients it is mandatory to perform TRUS followed by biopsy. If both PSA and DRE were positive, there was a 25% chance of finding a tumor if TRUS was considered normal; this figure increased to 83.9% if TRUS was positive. These figures are similar to those found by Lee et al. [16], who found a 71% chance of cancer when PSA, DRE and TRUS were positive.

In conclusion, figure 1 is an algorithm which we have worked out based upon our studies. When evaluating a patient with prostatic complaints, we routinely obtain a blood sample for PSA determination and perform a DRE; if they are both negative, we perform TRUS and a biopsy only in case of positive TRUS. If they are both positive, we perform TRUS and biopsy. If DRE is suspicious and PSA is normal or if DRE is normal and PSA is abnormal, we perform TRUS: if it is negative, we perform a random biopsy, while if it is positive, we perform an ultrasonically guided biopsy of the suspicious zone.

It is evident that even if we apply these studies skillfully, some clinically important prostate cancer will be missed. It is important that urologists inform patients that no procedure, or combination of them, available today will discover all cancers. However, it is sure that we may improve prostate cancer detection to a very significant degree by the judicious employment of these techniques. With this algorithm, we think we have reached a reasonable rate of false-positives and false-negatives.

## References


1 Holleb AI (ed): CA 1988 (Jan/Feb);38:5.
2 Guinan P, Bush I, Ray V, Vieth R, Rao R, Bhatti R: The accuracy of the rectal examination in the diagnosis of prostate carcinoma. N Engl J Med 1980;303:499.
3 Lee F, Littrup PJ, Torp-Pedersen ST: Screening for prostate cancer: comparison of transrectal ultrasound and the digital rectal examination. Radiology 1988;168:389.
4 Killian CS, Yang N, Emrich LJ: Prognostic importance of prostate-specific antigen for monitoring patients with stages B2 to D1 prostate cancer. Cancer Res 1985;45:886.
5 Cooner WH, Mosley BR, Rutherford CL Jr, Beard JH, Pond HS, Terry WJ, Igel TC, Kidd DD: Prostate cancer detection by ultrasonography, digital rectal examination and prostate-specific antigen. J Urol 1990;143:1146.
6 Lee F, Torp-Pedersen ST, Siders DB, Littrup PJ, McLeary RD: Transrectal ultrasound in the diagnosis and staging of prostatic carcinoma. Radiology 1989;170:609.
7 Cooner WH, Mosley BR, Rutherford CL Jr, Beard JH, Pond HS, Terry WJ, Igel TC, Kidd DD: Coordination of urosonography and prostate-specific antigen in the diagnosis of nonpalpable prostate cancer. J Endourol 1989;3:193.
8 Lee F, Littrup PJ, Torp-Pedersen ST, Mettlin C, McHugh TA, Gray JM, Kumasaka GH, McLeary RD: Prostate cancer: comparison of transrectal US and digital rectal examination for screening. Radiology 1988;168:389.
9 Oesterling JE: Prostate-specific antigen: a critical assessment of the most useful tumor marker for adenocarcinoma of the prostate. J Urol 1991;145:907.
10 Stamey TA, Yang N, Hay AR, McNeal JE, Freiha FS, Redwine E: Prostate-specific antigen as a serum marker for adenocarcinoma of the prostate. N Engl J Med 1987;317:909.
11 Oesterling JE, Chan DW, Epstein JI, Kimball AW, Bruzek DJ, Rock RC, Brendler CB, Walsh PC: Prostate-specific antigen in the preoperative and postoperative evaluation of localised prostatic cancer treated with radical prostatectomy. J Urol 1988;139:766.
12 Lindstedt G, Jacobsson A, Lundberg P, Hedelin H, Pettersson S, Unsgaard B: Determination of prostate-specific antigen in serum by immunoradiometric assay. Clin Chem 1988; 36:53.
13 Seamonds B, Yang N, Anderson K, Whitaker B, Shaw L, Bollinger JE: Evaluation of prostate-specific antigen and prostatic acid phosphatase as prostate cancer markers. Urology 1986;28:472.
14 Hudson MA, Bahnson RR, Catalona WJ: Clinical use of prostate-specific antigen in patients with prostate cancer. J Urol 1989;142:1011.
15 Lange PH, Ercole CJ, Lightner DJ, Fraley EE, Vessella R: The value of serum prostate specific antigen determinations before and after radical prostatectomy. J Urol 1989;141:873.
16 Lee F, Torp-Pedersen ST, Littrup PJ, McLeary RD, McHugh TA, Smid AP, Stella PJ, Borlaza GS: Hypoechoic lesions of the prostate: clinical relevance of tumor size, digital rectal examination and prostate-specific antigen. Radiology 1989;170:29.
17 Cooner WH: Prostate-specific antigen, digital rectal examination and transrectal ultrasonic examination of the prostate in prostate cancer detection. Monogr Urol 1991;12:3.
18 Cooner WH, Mosley BR, Rutherford CL: Clinical application of transrectal ultrasonography and PSA in the search for prostatic cancer. J Urol 1988;139:758.
19 Devonec M, Chapelon JY, Cathignol D: Comparison of the diagnostic value of sonography and rectal examination in cancer of the prostate. Eur Urol 1988;14:189.

Eur Urol 1992;21(suppl 1):92–95

*Franco Di Silverio*[a]
*Giuseppe D'Eramo*[a]
*Mauro Caponera*[a]
*Floriana Persechino*[a]
*Patrizia Eleuteri*[b]
*Delia Cavallo*[b]
*Raffaele De Vita*[b]
*Danilo Forte*[b]

[a] Department of Urology, University of Rome 'La Sapienza', and
[b] Environmental Biomedicine Division, ENEA, Casaccia, Rome, Italy

# The Prognostic Value of DNA Content in Patients with Prostatic Carcinoma

**Key Words**
Flow cytometry
Cellular ploidy
Prostate cancer

**Abstract**
In 80 patients with pathologically proven prostatic cancer, DNA content was correlated to grade, stage and survival. The survival curve and duration of response to therapy in these patients was examined. At the end of follow-up the cumulative survival curve in the aneuploid patients was 0.40, according to the Kaplan-Meier method, while in the diploid population it was 0.65. Differences between the two groups, aneuploid and diploid, were observed within the various histological subgroups: survival in the G2 population was 0.57 for the diploid and 0.30 for the aneuploid whereas in the G3 patients it was respectively 0.69 for the diploid and 0.05 for the aneuploid patients.

## Introduction

Prostate cancer is the most common malignant tumor in men [1]. During the past years the advent of new diagnostic tools has increased the incidence of early diagnosis, but the inability to predict prostatic cancer's clinical outcome, due to the disease's extremely variable natural history [2], remains a dilemma in patient management. In numerous studies the following variables have been used in an attempt to accurately determine tumor aggressiveness: clinical and pathological stage, histological grade, nuclear and nucleolar morphology, tumor volume, steroid hormone receptors, prostate acid phosphatase (PAP) and prostate-specific antigen (PSA) [3–13]. The parameters most often used are tumor grade and stage, this last one however cannot be considered as objective.

Currently, nuclear morphology and cytofluorometry have taken on increased significance due to their objective nature, repeatability and quantitability. Furthermore, molecular biology studies of the genome in prostatic cancer seem to indicate the importance of deletions on the short arm of chromosomes 8 and 10 and on the long arm of chromosome 16 [14, 15].

Our major aim remains that of being able to accurately determine the individual patient's prognosis, in early or later stages of the disease, and its metastatic potential in order to effectively program treatment. The aim of this study was the evaluation of cellular DNA ploidy as an indicator of prognosis in patients with prostatic carcinoma.

## Materials and Methods

*Patients*

One hundred and eleven patients, average age 66.7 years (range 43–86), with pathologically proven prostatic cancer were initially recruited; in 80 of these patients, histological grade according to

Prof. Franco Di Silverio
Dipartimento di Urologia U. Bracci
Università degli Studi di Roma La Sapienza
Policlinico Umberto I, Viale del Policlinico
I-00161 Roma (Italy)


0302–2838/92/0215–0092
$2.75/0

Mostofi [16], cellular ploidy and PSA values during treatment were available for evaluation. Follow-up periods ranged from 54 to 102 months. Survival curves were calculated using the Kaplan-Meier product limit method [17].

*Samples*

Transperineal biopsy of the prostate with a Tru-Cut biopsy needle under sonographic guidance was performed and multiple specimens from both lobes, apex and base were obtained, according to Hodge's technique [18]. These samples were used for histological classification according to Mostofi [16] and flow cytometry analysis.

The samples for flow cytometric analysis were stored at 4 °C in RPMI 1640 medium (Gibco, New York, N.Y., USA) supplemented with 5% fetal calf serum. First, the samples were washed in physiological solution (0.9% NaCl). Monocellular suspensions were obtained by mechanical treatment with scissors [19]. The cellular suspensions were fixed with 70% ethanol and stored at 4 °C. Part of the specimens were also used for cytologic examination in an attempt to verify their quality for cytometric measurements.

*Flow Cytometry Staining*

The fixed samples were centrifuged at 200 *g* for 10 min, and the pellets were resuspended in 5% pepsin solution (pH 1.8) for 10 min at room temperature, under continuous gentle magnetic stirring. The pepsin was then neutralized with 0.1 *M* Tris buffer solution; the samples were centrifuged under the same conditions as before, and the pellets resuspended in the same buffer. The cells were finally stained with a dye solution containing 5 mg/ml ethidium bromide (Serva), 12.5 mg/ml mitramycin (Pfizer Inc., New York N.Y., USA), and 7.5 m*M* $MgCl_2$ in 0.1 *M* Tris buffer (pH 7.4) filtered through a 70-nm nylon mesh, and kept at 4 °C for 30–60 min before flow cytometric analysis [19].

*Flow Cytometry*

The samples were analyzed with a PAS II flow cytometer (Partec, Arlesheim, Switzerland). The signals were collected and accumulated on a 512-channel memory. The histograms were stored on a floppy disk and analyzed by an original software protocol on a PC-XT IBM personal computer. Flow cytometric analysis was performed according to the recommendations suggested for DNA cytometry nomenclature [20]. For each case analyzed, the lymphocytes or a normal prostate cell sample of the same patient was used as an external and internal standard of cytometrically diploid DNA content [21]. Samples exhibiting one or more subpopulations with abnormal DNA content were defined as cytometrically aneuploid. The level of DNA content alteration was expressed in terms of DNA index (DI), calculated as the ratio of the G1/0 modal values between the aneuploid and diploid subpopulations. The analysis of DNA histogram data to calculate the cell cycle frequencies (%G1/O, %S1, %G2+M) was performed by a cumulative curve graphic method [20] elaborated by software developed in our laboratory according to the method proposed by Baisch et al. [22].

*Follow-Up*

Transrectal ultrasonography with a 7-MHz probe was performed for the evaluation of local extension, whereas for the determination of lymph node status, computerized tomography and nuclear magnetic resonance was used, and total body bone scans, abdominal ultrasonography and a plain film of the chest for the determination of eventual metastases.

RIA, testosterone, LH, FSH, PAP and PSA values were determined before beginning therapy and afterwards for every 3 months. Treatment consisted in the use of LHRH analogue alone or in combination with cyproterone acetate.

## Results

Patients were staged according to the AUS classification. Clinically, 6 patients were stage A-B, 4 (66.6%) diploid and 2 (33.4%) aneuploid; 18 patients stage $C_1$, 12 (66.6%) diploid and 6 (33.4%) aneuploid; 19 patients were stage $C_2$, 12 (63.2%) diploid and 7 (36.8%) aneuploid. 3 (42.8%) out of 7 $D_1$ patients were diploid, while 4 (57.2%) were aneuploid; 11 (36.6%) out of 30 $D_2$ patients showed a diploid pattern, while 19 (63.3%) had an aneuploid pattern.

According to the grading and cellular ploidy, 16 patients (20%) were G1, 14 (87.5%) diploid and 2 (12.5%) aneuploid; 38 G2 (47.5%), 21 (55.3%) diploid and 17 (44.7%) aneuploid; 26 (32.5%) G3, 7 (29.9%) diploid and 19 (73.1%) aneuploid.

The patients with a grade 1 and 2 prostate carcinoma showed the same survival curve, with 52 and 45% of survival after 60 months of follow-up. The survival of G3 patients decreased rapidly from 45 to 5% in the follow-up period and ranged from 40 and 48 months (fig. 1).

If we consider the survival related to the cellular ploidy, the better value is that of diploid patients, with a value of 65% after 60 months; the aneuploid patient survival was 40% after the same follow-up period (fig. 2).

The survival of patients with the same histological grade was studied in relation to cytometric ploidy with the Kaplan-Meier method. In the G1 group the survival was the same for diploid and aneuploid patients, also considering the low number of aneuploid patients in this group. In the G2 group, survival was 57% for the diploid and 30% for the aneuploid patients, with a not statistically significant difference (fig. 3). In the G3 group, survival values were respectively 45% for the diploid and 5% for the aneuploid patients, with a statistically significant difference ($p < 0.05$) between the two groups (fig. 4). Our data confirmed the higher percentage of aneuploid pattern in patients with advanced disease and higher grade (fig. 5, 6). Analysis of cellular DNA content of prostatic carcinomas by flow cytometry has revealed a significantly higher proportion ($<0.05$) of aneuploidy in advanced stages (C–D) and a similar correlation to loss of tumor differentiation (G grading), while no significant correlation between ploidy and T stage was observed.

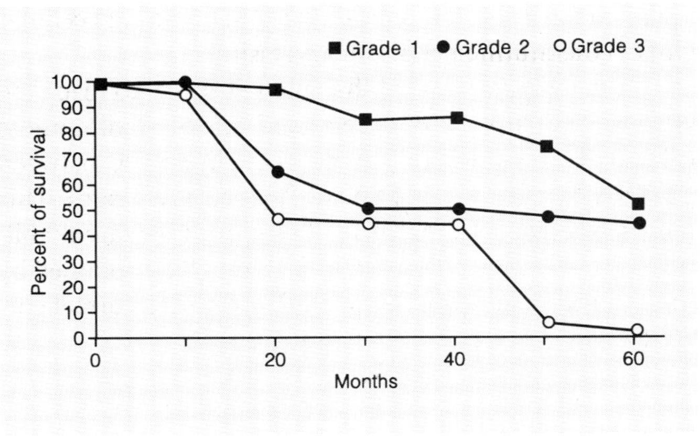


**Fig. 1.** Cumulative survival curve versus grade in patients with prostatic carcinoma.

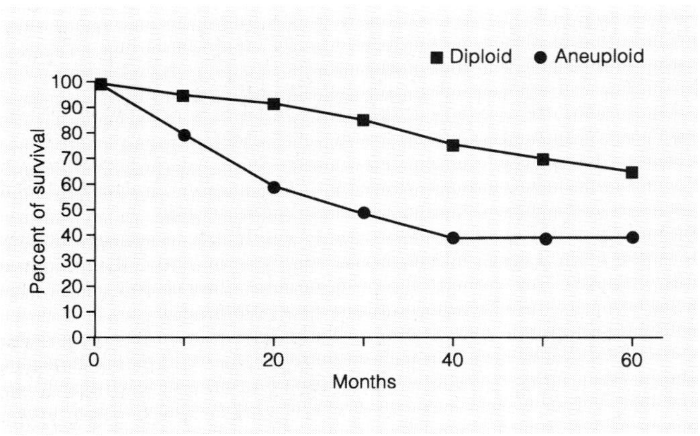


**Fig. 2.** Cumulative survival curve versus ploidy in patients with prostatic carcinoma.

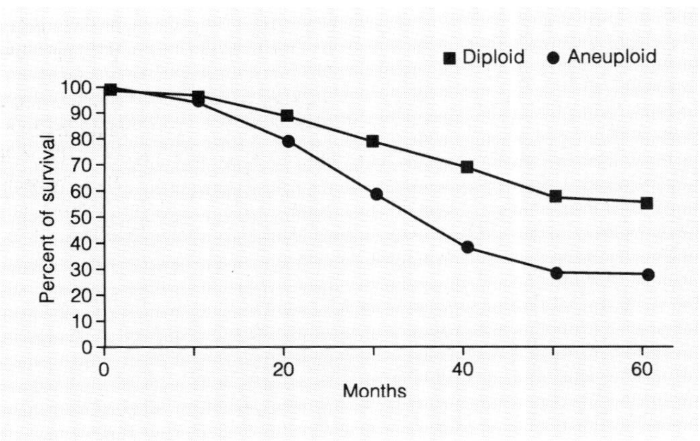


**Fig. 3.** Survival versus ploidy in G2 patients.

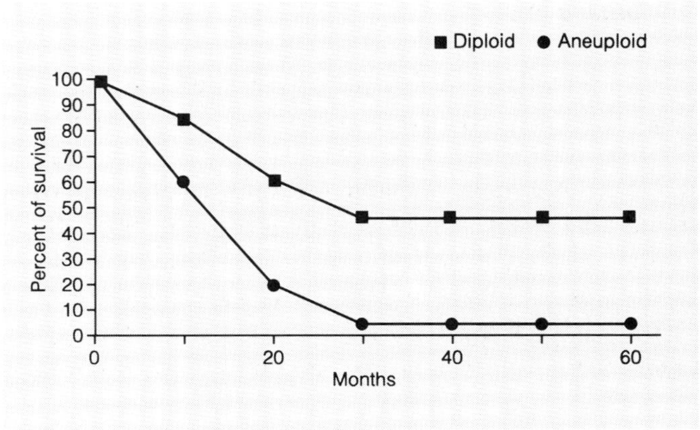


**Fig. 4.** Survival versus ploidy in G3 patients.

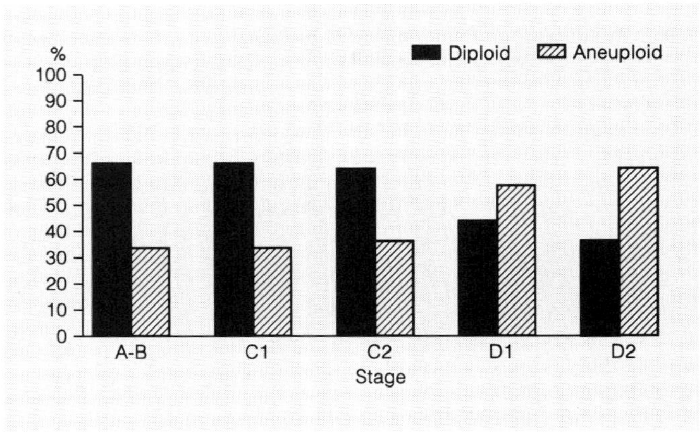


**Fig. 5.** Ploidy versus staging in patients with prostatic carcinoma.

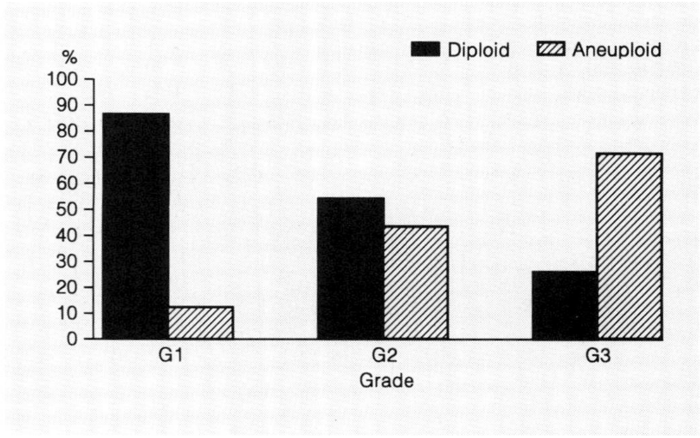


**Fig. 6.** Ploidy versus grading in patients with prostatic carcinoma.

## Conclusions

For the urologist it is always more useful to obtain an early diagnosis because of the increasing incidence of prostatic carcinoma. To reach this goal, with the improving of technological procedures, results in better choice of proper therapy. A deeper knowledge of the features which may affect the disease's development and their prognostic factor values allows for more reliable therapy and decision-making. In the evaluation parameters, cellular DNA content by flow cytometry on the surgical specimens seems to result in a possible discrimination of the cellular clones constituting neoplasm aggression.

The predictive value of this method seems to reach the best reliability in undifferentiated histological tumors (G3), with a statistically significant difference between diploid and aneuploid patients about survival rates. This parameter did not succeed in obtaining an equal reliability in G1 tumor patients. Better results will be obtained by the analysis of a higher number of cases and a correct correlation with other prognostic factors.

## References


1 Silverberg E, Lubera JA: Cancer statistics, 1989. Cancer 1989;39:3.
2 Whitmore WF Jr: The natural history and staging of prostatic cancer. Urol Clin North Am 1984;11:205.
3 Gleason DF, Mellinger GT, Veterans Administration Cooperative Urological Research Group: Prediction of prognosis for prostatic adenocarcinoma by combined histological grading and clinical staging. J Urol 1974;11: 58–64.
4 Partin AW, Walsch AC, Pitcock RV, Mohler JL, Epstein JI, Coffey DS: A comparison of nuclear morphometry and Gleason grade as a predictor of prognosis in stage A2 prostate cancer: a critical analysis. J Urol 1989;142:1254–1258.
5 Petrangeli E, Ferraro F, Di Giovanni L, Marocchi A, Sciarra F, Di Silverio F, Toscano V, Concolino G: Homogenization buffers and subcellular distribution of androgen receptors and endogenous DHT in human prostate tissue. (abstract). 3rd Int Forum of Andrology, Paris 1985, p 17.
6 Nativ O, Myers RP, Farrow G, Therneau TM, Zincke H, Lieber MM: Nuclear deoxyribonucleic acid ploidy and serum prostate-specific antigen in operable prostatic carcinoma. J Urol 1990;144:303–306.
7 Miller J, Horsfall DJ, Marshall DM, Rao DM, Leong SY: The prognostic value of deoxyribonucleic acid flow cytometry analysis in stage D2 prostatic cancer. J Urol 1991;145:1192–1196.
8 Di Silverio F, Tenaglia R, Devita R, De Matteis A: Valutazione clinica del rapporto tra ploidia citometrica e grading delle neoplasie urologiche. Acta Urol Ital 1987;1:17–19.
9 Winkler HZ, Rainwater LM, Myers RP, Farrow GM, Therneau TM, Zincke H, Lieber MM: Stage D1 prostatic adenocarcinoma: significance of nuclear DNA ploidy patterns studied by flow cytometry. Mayo Clin Proc 1988; 63:103–112.
10 Winkler HZ, Rainwater LM, Myers RP, Farrow GM, Therneau TM, Zincke H, Lieber MM, Nativ O, Raz Y, Hosaka Y, Boyle ET: Prognostic significance of DNA ploidy in stage C and D1 prostate cancer. J Urol 1991;145: abstr 698.
11 Greene DR, Taylor SR, Wheeler TM, Scardino PT: DNA ploidy analysis of incidental and early prostate cancer. J Urol 1991;142:abstr 746.
12 Nagel R, Al-Abadi H: The prognostic significance of ploidy and DNA heterogeneity in the primary diagnosis and monitoring of patients with locally advanced prostatic carcinoma. Scand J Urol Nephrol 1991;138(suppl):83–92.
13 Blute ML, Nativ O, Zincke H, Farrow GM, Therneau T, Lieber MM: Pattern of failure after radical retropubic prostatectomy for clinically and pathologically localized adenocarcinoma of the prostate: influence of tumor deoxyribonucleic acid ploidy. J Urol 1989;142: 1262–1265.
14 Bergerheim USR, Collins VP, Ekman P, Kunimi K: Recessive genetic mechanisms in the oncogenesis of prostatic carcinoma. Scand J Urol Nephrol 1991;138(suppl):93–96.
15 Carter BS, Ewing CM, Ward WS, Treiger BF, Aalders TW, Schalken JA, Epstein JI, Issacs WB: Allelic loss of chromosomes 16q and 10q in human prostate cancer. Proc Natl Acad Sci USA 1990;87:8751–8755.
16 Mostofi FK: Grading of prostatic carcinoma. Cancer Chemother Rep 1975;59:111–117.
17 Kaplan EL, Meier P: Nonparametric estimation from incomplete observations. J Am Stat Assoc 1958;53:457–481.
18 Hodge KK, McNeal JE, Terris MK, Stamey TA: Random systematic versus directed ultrasound guided transrectal core biopsies of the prostate. J Urol 1989;142:71–75.
19 Zante J, Schumann J, Barlogie B: New preparation and staining procedures for rapid analysis of DNA distribution; in Ghode W, Schumann J, Buchner T (eds): Second International Symposium on Pulse Cytophotometry, Ghent, European Press Medikon, 1976, pp 97–106.
20 Hiddemann W, Schumann J, Andreff M: Convention on nomenclature of DNA cytometry. Cytometry 1984;5:445–446.
21 Gohnde W, Schumann J, Buchner T: Pulse cytometry: Application in tumor cell biology and clinical oncology; in Melamed MR, Mullaney IF, Mendelsohn MI (eds): Flow Cytometry and Sorting. New York, Wiley, 1979, pp 599–620.
22 Baisch H, Gohnde W, Linden WA: Mathematical analysis of ICP data to determine the fraction of cells in the various phases of the cell cycle; in Haanen CAM, Hiller HFO, Wessels JMC (eds): 1st Int Symp on Pulse Cytophotometry. Ghent, European Press Medikon, 1975, pp 68–76.

Eur Urol 1992;21(suppl 1):96–98

*G. Zanetti*
*A. Trinchieri*
*A. Del Nero*
*E. Montanari*
*M. Cogni*
*F. Colombo*
*V. Buzzetti*
*E. Austoni*

Institute of Urology (Head: Prof. *E. Pisani*), University of Milan, Italy

# Prognostic Significance of Prostate-Specific Antigen in Endocrine Treatment for Prostatic Carcinoma

**Key Words**
Prostatic cancer
Prostate-specific antigen
Endocrine treatment

**Abstract**
We have studied the prognostic significance of prostate-specific antigen (PSA), monitored monthly, in 24 patients with prostatic cancer (5 D1, 19 D2) on endocrine therapy. The pretreatment levels of PSA were high in all patients (mean value 41 ng/ml). It was found that PSA levels at the end of the first and sixth months of treatment were reliable prognostic indicators. At the first month evaluation PSA had decreased more than 50% from the initial values in the 16 patients with stable disease, while it had decreased less than 50% in those with progressing disease. At the end of 6 months, patients with stable disease had PSA levels within the normal range, while 8 of the patients who had progressing disease had levels higher than 10 ng/ml. Respectively 6 and 2 patients had also had increases in PSA levels at 3 and 6 months before scintigraphic demonstration of increased bone metastases.

## Introduction

Prostate-specific antigen (PSA), identified and purified for the first time in 1979, is a glycoprotein produced exclusively by the acinar and ductal epithelial cells of the prostate gland. From the earliest clinical studies, PSA has been found to be a more sensitive diagnostic marker for prostatic carcinoma than prostatic acid phosphatase (PAP). Myrtle et al. [1], in a review in 1986 of 553 patients with prostatic carcinoma, found levels of PSA above the upper limit of normal in 81% of cases, with associated similar increases in PAP in only 43% of cases. Kuriyama et al. [2], Ahmann and Schifman [3] and Arai et al. [4] all showed the usefulness of PSA determinations in monitoring responses to hormonal treatment, with PSA increasing with progression of the disease. However, Leo et al. [5] compared PSA levels of two groups of patients with stage D2 disease, the first group on antiandrogen treatment and the second without previous hormone treatment, and found a positive direct effect of androgen deprivation on plasma PSA levels which was independent from the response to treatment. For these reasons, we have studied the prognostic reliability of PSA for patients with advanced prostatic carcinoma being treated with hormones.

## Materials and Methods

PSA before treatment was measured in 24 patients, 5 with clinical stage D1 and 19 with clinical stage D2 disease. The mean age was 68 years, range 48–81 years. Pretreatment staging was based on clinical examination, chest X-ray, urography, upper and lower abdominal

Dr. Gian Paolo Zanetti
Istituto di Urologia, Università di Milano
Via della Commenda, 15
I-20100 Milano (Italy)


0302–2838/92/0215–0096
$2.75/0

CT, bone scintigraphy and transrectal prostatic ultrasonography. None of the patients had been given any endocrine treatment nor other treatments such as radiotherapy or disobstructive TURP. All the patients were treated with the depot preparation of a luteinizing-releasing hormone (LHRH) agonist (goserelin). For follow-up, PSA was determined every month. Every 3 months, blood chemistry and complete hormone analyses were done, along with transrectal prostatic ultrasonography and bone scintigraphy. Every 6 months, chest X-rays and abdominal pelvic CT were obtained.

The serum samples were obtained before any manipulation of the prostate gland, separated from the blood within 2–3 h of collection and stored frozen at –20 °C. Serum PSA was measured by the Milenia PSA (EURO/DPC Ltd), a kinetic enzyme immunometric assay, according to the manufacturer's instructions. In brief, patient's samples are added to ligand-coated wells, along with a master reagent consisting of both ligand-labeled and horseradish peroxidase-labeled monoclonal antibodies specific for PSA. During the initial 30-min reaction, endogenous PSA reacts with the monoclonal antibodies in liquid phase. During a second 30-min incubation the addition of multivalent antiligand creates a bridge between the PSA/anti-PSA complexes and the ligand-coated wells. The microplate is then washed to remove unreacted material. A chromogenic substrate that reacts with the enzyme label is then added, and the rate of color development is ascertained using a kinetic microplate analyzer during a 5-min reading period at 450 nm. Reaction rates are directly related to endogenous PSA concentrations.

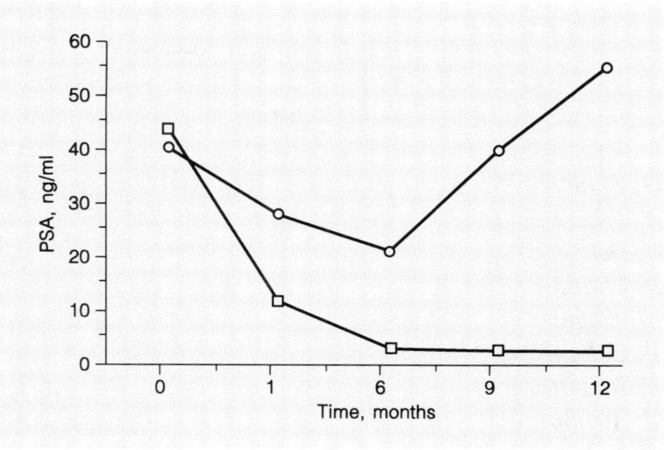


**Fig. 1.** PSA levels in endocrine treatment during 1 year of follow-up (n = 24). □ = Patients with stable disease (n = 16); ○ = patients with progressing disease (n = 8).

## Results

Pretreatment PSA levels were found to be higher than normal values in all 24 patients, with a mean value of 41 ng/ml (range 9.5–70.7). The pretreatment levels of PSA were then analyzed in relation to the interval free of progression. The patients were divided into two groups: group 1 (6 patients) had PSA $<30$ ng/ml and group 2 (18 patients) had PSA $>30$ ng/ml. We observed no significant difference in progression-free duration in the two groups. PSA levels were significantly decreased in all patients 1 month after the start of treatment. The magnitude of the decrease was found to be a reliable prognostic factor for the response to endocrine treatment. PSA levels in the 16 patients whose diseases were stable 1 year after the start of treatment had decreased more than 50%, while they had decreased less than 50% in the 8 patients whose diseases had progressed ($p = 0.016$) (fig. 1). Particularly, in the group with stable disease, PSA demonstrated a variation from basal levels of $42.04 \pm 17.28$ to $10.26 \pm 6.79$ ng/ml (mean $\pm$ SD) ($p < 0.0001$), while in the group that had progressing disease the observed variation was from $38.95 \pm 12.98$ to $26.26 \pm 9.64$ ng/ml (mean $\pm$ SD) ($p < 0.0001$). PSA levels after 6 months of treatment were also reliable prognostically. The 16 patients with stable disease had PSA within the limits of normal (0.1–3.5 ng/ml), while the other 8 patients had levels higher than 10 ng/ml. The serial determinations of PSA were then analyzed for the 8 patients with progressive disease in relation to the areas of high tracer uptake in bone scintigraphy. Six patients had increases in PSA levels 3 months before scintigraphy could demonstrate the bone metastases, and 2 had increases about 6 months before the scintigrams became positive.

## Discussion

Until about 10 years ago, the only marker for prostatic carcinoma was PAP, a ubiquitous enzyme that is not specific to prostatic tissue, difficult to assay because of interference by the isoenzymes produced in other organs with measurement of the isoenzyme produced specifically in the prostatic tissue. The discovery of PSA, produced only by acinar and ductal epithelial cells of the prostate gland, was hailed with enthusiasm because it might be used to diagnose and to monitor prostatic cancer during treatment. On the basis of the data in the literature, the most promising role of PSA appears to be monitoring of the disease during treatment, especially for evaluation of residual disease after radical prostatectomy. There has been less investigation of the reliability of monitoring PSA during hormonal treatment. Recent experiences [5–8] have indicated that there is a direct effect of antiandrogen treatment on expression of PSA, an effect that is independent of the antitumor effect of the antiandrogens.

In spite of this, our trial indicates that PSA is a reliable prognostic indicator during follow-up of prostatic carcinoma. Pretreatment levels of PSA are not significantly correlated with the response to endocrine treatment, but PSA levels at the end of 1 month of treatment, and even more the percentage decrease from the basal values, can be used to predict response to treatment, the duration of which can be estimated with sufficient reliability on the basis of the PSA levels at 6 months: patients with PSA values within the range of normal have a high probability of prolonged responses, while patients with levels higher than 10 ng/ml should be expected to progress.

## References


1 Myrtle JF, Klimley PG, Ivor LP, Brun JF: Clinical utility of prostate-specific antigen in the management of prostate cancer. Adv Cancer Diag, San Diego, Hybritech Inc, 1986.

2 Kuriyama M, Wang MC, Lee CL, Papsidero LD, Killian CS, Inaji H, Slack NH, Nishiura T, Murphy GP, Chu TM: Use of human prostate-specific antigen in monitoring prostate cancer. Cancer Res 1981;4:3874–3876.

3 Ahmann FR, Schifman RB: Prospective comparison between serum monoclonal prostate-specific antigen and acid phosphatase measurement in metastatic prostate cancer. J Urol 1987;137:431–434.

4 Arai Y, Yoshiki T, Yoshida O: Prognostic significance of prostate-specific antigen in endocrine treatment for prostatic cancer. J Urol 1990;144:1415–1418.

5 Leo ME, Bilhartz DL, Bergstralh E, Oesterling JE: Prostate-specific antigen in hormonally treated stage D2 prostate cancer: Is it always an accurate indicator of disease status? J Urol 1991;145:802–806.

6 Stamey TA, Kabalin JN, Ferrari M, Yang N: Prostate-specific antigen in the diagnosis and treatment of adenocarcinoma of the prostate. IV. Anti-androgen treated patients. J Urol 1989;141:1088–1090.

7 Weber JP, Oesterling JE, Peters CA, Partin AW, Chan DW, Walsh PC: The influence of reversible androgen deprivation on serum prostate-specific antigen levels in men with benign prostatic hyperplasia. J Urol 1989;141: 987–992.

8 Csapo Z, Brand K, Walther R, Fokas K: Comparative experimental study of the serum prostate-specific antigen and prostatic acid phosphatase in serially transplantable human prostatic carcinoma lines in nude mice. J Urol 1988;140:1032–1038.

Eur Urol 1992;21(suppl 1):99–101

*F. Zattoni*
*R. Piazza*
*R. Vianello*
*A. Garbeglio*
*F. Pagano*

Institute of Urology, Padua University, Padua, Italy

# Preoperative and Postoperative Evaluation of Prostate-Specific Antigen in Localized Prostatic Cancer Treated by Radical Prostatectomy

**Key Words**
Prostatic carcinoma
Prostate-specific antigen
Radical prostatectomy

**Abstract**
Preoperative prostate-specific antigen (PSA) values were determined in 73 patients with clinically localized prostatic cancer and candidates for a radical procedure. Correlation of preoperative PSA with a final pathological stage was attempted. Only in 44.8% of our 22 patients with organ-confined disease was the PSA value within the normal range; in 17.3% of cases PSA values were higher than 20 ng/ml. 18.2% of the patients with locally advanced disease showed normal PSA values, while 45.5% had concentrations above 20 ng/ml. In the case of lymph node involvement, PSA values were normal in 22.7% of the cases. Our data indicate that no strict relationship can be suggested between PSA and the final pathological stage and grading of the tumor in patients who underwent radical prostatectomy.

## Introduction

Several clinical studies have shown that prostate-specific disease (PSA) is an effective marker to monitor patients with advanced prostatic cancer [1–3]. A direct correlation between PSA levels and the clinical course of the patient was even observed [3]. Almost invariably as the tumor progresses serum PSA concentration increases, and as the cancer regresses during therapy, PSA levels also decrease steadily [3–5]. Concerning the significance and the utility of PSA concentrations in patients with localized prostatic cancer, just recently Oesterling et al. [2] investigated the ability of PSA to predict the final pathological stage in patients with clinically localized prostatic cancer prior to radical prostatectomy.

In this report we review our experience on serum determination of PSA in a group of patients who underwent subsequent radical prostatectomy.

## Materials

From February 1986 to December 1990, in 73 previously untreated patients with clinically localized prostatic cancer and candidates for a radical procedure, preoperative serum PSA was determined using the Tandem-R PSA monoclonal immunoradiometric assay.

Patients underwent bilateral staging pelvic lymphadenectomy and radical retropubic prostatectomy. Based on the final pathological findings, all patients were divided into three categories: (a) with organ-confined disease (pathological stage B disease); (b) with capsular penetration and/or seminal vesicle involvement (stage C cancer),

Dr. Filiberto Zattoni
Istituto di Urologia, Università di Padova
Via Giustiniani, 2
I-35100 Padova (Italy)


0302–2838/92/0215–0099
$2.75/0

**Table 1.** Correlation between pathological stage and preoperative PSA serum values (n = 73)

| Pathological stage | PSA, ng/ml | | | | Patients |
|---|---|---|---|---|---|
| | <4 | 4–10 | 10.1–20 | >20 | |
| B | 13 (44.8%) | 8 (27.6%) | 3 (10.3%) | 5 (17.3%) | 29 |
| C | 4 (18.2%) | 1 (4.5%) | 7 (31.8%) | 10 (45.5%) | 22 |
| D1 | 5 (22.7%) | 4 (18.2%) | 6 (27.3%) | 7 (31.8%) | 22 |

**Table 2.** Correlation between preoperative PSA serum values and Gleason score

| Gleason score | PSA, ng/ml | | | | Patients |
|---|---|---|---|---|---|
| | <4 | 4–10 | 10.1–20 | >20 | |
| 2–4 | 6 | 2 | 1 | 1 | 10 |
| 5–7 | 11 | 6 | 12 | 9 | 38 |
| 8–10 | 5 | 5 | 3 | 12 | 25 |

and (c) with lymph node invasion (D1 cancer). Correlation of preoperative PSA with final pathological stage was attempted.

Separate analysis was performed for each final pathologic stage and for four different concentrations (ng/ml) of PSA value (<4, 4–10, 10.1–20, >20). Comparative analysis was even done between histological grading (according to the Gleason system) and different PSA concentration categories.

PSA concentrations were also evaluated between the third and fifth days in the immediate postoperative period. Postoperative long-term follow-up with periodical PSA dosage is also available for 41 patients: the period between radical surgery and measurement of the postoperative PSA ranged from 6 to 61 months (mean 33.6).

## Results

Using the Tandem-R PSA assay, the upper limit of the normal range for men without prostatic disease is considered to be 4.0 ng/ml. From our experience it resulted that 13 (44.8%) of the 29 patients with organ-confined disease presented preoperative PSA values included in the normal range. Only 5 cases (17.3%) had values >20 ng/ml (table 1).

Four (18.2%) of the 22 patients with locally advanced cancer showed normal ranges of PSA values; 10 cases (45.5%) had concentrations >20 ng/ml. In the case of lymph node involvement however, in 5 (22.7%) cases out of 22 patients normal PSA values were discovered preoperatively; 7 cases (31.8%) had values >20 ng/ml.

In table 2, results coming from the comparison of PSA with different histological categories are presented. With values of PSA >20 ng/ml and the Gleason score between 8 and 10 the possibility to discover an organ-confined disease cannot be excluded.

The PSA dosages at the third and fifth postoperative days demonstrated a significant reduction superior to the two-thirds of the initial values. In the short-term follow-up only 4 patients (5.7%) continued to have persistent elevated values of PSA after a range of 30–90 days. One case (stage C2 disease) with persistent abnormal PSA values presented evidence of recurrent disease 8 months after surgery.

## Discussion

From our series of patients it results that 51 (69.8%) of 73 of all the candidates for a radical prostatectomy presented serum PSA values variably above the upper normal level. Vice versa, in 9 (40.9%) of the 22 patients with normal PSA values, a locally extended tumor or a nodal extension was found. It derives that, contrary to others' experience [2], normal PSA concentrations were compatible even with lymph nodal invasion. Normal PSA values reflected an organ-confined disease in only 13 patients (17.8% of the entire number). A large spread of values was noted for each pathological category, as well as for each histological grading. Even if the highest PSA concentrations were found in locally advanced tumors and in cases with nodal involvement, no relationship can be suggested between PSA and histological grading. In patients who underwent radical prostatectomy, persistent abnormal values of PSA are commonly considered as an indicator of incomplete tumor excision with severe changes of presenting clinically recurrence of disease in longer follow-up [1]. Oesterling et al. [2] found that 3.15 ± 0.09 days is the half-life time for PSA. This consideration is relevant as it allows to know whether the PSA measured on the postoperative period reflects the presence of tumor left behind or a normally decreasing serum titer after removal of all prostatic tissue. Such a parameter has to be seriously considered in the decision for eventual adjuvant therapy and for time of starting it.

## Conclusion

PSA must be considered a sensitive biochemical marker to follow patients after radical prostatectomy. Periodical evaluation is required in order to detect eventual modifications of the marker which should ideally be maintained within the female range. In the experience of Oesterling et al. [2] all patients with clinical recurrence, either local or distant, had an elevated serum PSA concentration. On the contrary, PSA as an isolated marker does not appear to be useful in preoperative prediction of the final pathological stage of the prostatic cancer on the individual basis due to the large spread of values [3]. Even the association with the tumor grading does not improve the possibility of any individual prediction on the pathological stage [6].

In metastatic cancer it has been largely demonstrated that elevated pretreatment PSA values would indicate poorer prognosis and shorter survival [4–7]. High preoperative PSA concentrations in patient candidates for radical prostatectomy, which return into the normal ranges within a few days after surgery, are probably related to the tumor bulk which is even conditioning the possibility of distant metastases [8]. At present we do not have any answer on the future clinical and biological significance of these abnormal preoperative PSA values. On the contrary, persistent abnormal PSA values after radical prostatectomy which do not follow the normal half-time decrease certainly represent a negative prognostic factor in the long-term follow-up.

## References


1 Hudson MA, Bahnson RR, Catalona WJ: Clinical use of specific antigen in patients with prostate cancer. J Urol 1989;142:1011–1017.
2 Oesterling JE, Chan DW, Epstein JI, Kimball AW, Bruzek DJ, Rock RC, Brendler CB, Walsh PC: Prostate-specific antigen in the preoperative and postoperative evaluation of localized prostatic cancer treated with radical prostatectomy. J Urol 1988;139:766–772.
3 Kuriyama M, Wang MC, Lee CI, Papsidern LD, Killian CS, Inaji H, Slack NH, Nishiura T, Murphy GP, Chu TM: Use of human prostate-specific antigen in monitoring prostate cancer. Cancer Res 1981;41:3874.
4 Killian CR, Emrich LJ, Constantine R, Wang MC, Chu MT: Prognostic importance of PSA and other markers for monitoring of prostate cancer patients; in Tumor Marker in Prostate Cancer. Symp Proc. New York, Excepta Medica, 1986, pp 24–36.
5 Zattoni F, Oliva G, Piazza R, Vianello F, Maruzzi D, Pagano F: Esperienza con LHRH analoghi: valutazione della risposta clinica in relazione ad alcuni parametri di laboratorio. Acta Urol Ital 1988;4(suppl 1):59–63.
6 Zattoni F, Oliva G, Piazza R, Vianello F, Pagano F: La stadiazione clinica della neoplasia prostatica: limiti e prospettive. 61 Congresso Nazionale SIU, Cagliari 1988. Acta Urol Ital 1989;4(suppl 1):409–410.
7 Killian CS, Yang N, Emrich LJ, et al: Prognostic importance of PSA for monitoring patients with stage B2 to D1 prostate cancer. Cancer Res 1985;45:886–891.
8 Kahalin JN, Mc Neal JF, Price HM, Freiha FS, Stamey TA: Unsuspected adenocarcinoma of the prostate in patients undergoing cystoprostatectomy for other causes: incidence, histology and morphometric observation. J Urol 1989; 141/5:1091–1094.

Eur Urol 1992;21(suppl 1):102–104

*M. Marcellini*[a]
*P. De Carli*[a]
*M.R. Abbolito*[b]
*G. Mainiero*[a]
*R. Cantiani*[a]

[a] Division of Urology and
[b] Laboratory of Clinical Analyses,
Regina Elena National Cancer Institute,
Rome, Italy

# Serum Osteocalcin in Monitoring Bone Metastases in Advanced Prostatic Cancer

**Key Words**
Serum osteocalcin
Prostatic carcinoma
Tumor markers

**Abstract**
Osteocalcin, a K-dependent vitamin protein, was studied in a group of advanced prostatic carcinoma patients to test the usefulness of this marker for diagnosing bone metastases. Osteocalcin levels were above the norm in 22 out of 27 patients with bone metastases, although high levels were not observed in patients without bone metastases. High sensitivity and specificity levels of serum osteocalcin appear to be strongly correlated to metastatic bone involvement and disease relapse after hormone treatment. Although these results must be confirmed on a larger series of patients, this protein appears to be a useful biological marker in prostatic cancer.

## Introduction

Osteocalcin, a K-dependent vitamin protein that originates exclusively from bone tissue, plays an important role in phosphocalcic homeostasis. It increases the reactivity of osteoblasts and may therefore be a valuable marker of bone metastases in prostatic carcinoma.

The present study was conducted to evaluate the value of osteocalcin in the diagnosis and skeletal monitoring of advanced prostatic carcinoma patients. These levels were measured with a radioimmunological method at the time of the clinical diagnosis and then every 3 months during the course of hormone therapy. The sensitivity and specificity of osteocalcin for evaluating skeletal involvement of bone metastases in prostate cancer have been examined and discussed.

## Materials and Methods

Fifty-two patients with advanced prostatic carcinoma between the ages of 65 and 79 years were observed in the Division of Urology of the Regina Elena National Cancer Institute. Twenty-five were classified as stage C and 27 as stage D with grades G1 to G2 (according to Mostofi). Clinical staging was carried out by means of normal diagnostic radiographic and laboratory tests. Radiographic and scintigraphic examinations were used to evaluate the skeleton and the osteolytic-, osteoblastic- or mixed-type metastastic aspects.

At diagnosis, the following markers were evaluated in all of the patients: serum osteocalcin, PAP and PSA. The osteocalcin levels were evaluated by means of a radioimmunological method (OSCA-test Osteocalcin RIA; Henning Berlin GmbH), the normal values in our laboratory ranging between 4 and 10 ng/ml. The markers were measured at the start of the hormone treatment, consisting of an LHRH analogue and flutamide and then at 3-months intervals during treatment.

Dr. Mario Marcellini
Divisione di Urologia, Istituto Regina Elena
Viale Regina Elena, 291
I-00161 Roma (Italy)


0302–2838/92/0215–0102
$2.75/0

## Results

The markers evaluated at the time of diagnosis showed high PSA and PAP values both in patients with bone metastases as well as in those without. Osteocalcin levels, instead, were above the norm in 22 out of 27 patients with bone metastases and in no case in the absence of metastases (table 1).

Then monitored during hormone therapy, the osteocalcin levels tended to become normal, parallel with the clinical response in patients with bone metastases (table 2). In fact, these values returned to normal in 13 patients, the same patients in whom the disappearance of the bone pain was supported by regression of the radiological and/or scintigraphic findings. On the other hand, the PSA and PAP values during treatment did not follow the course of the bone metastases in the same specific manner, but did decrease.

During follow-up, the osteocalcin increases revealed the appearance of bone metastases, even during therapy in 8 cases (table 3). These metastases, revealed at scintigraphy and later radiologically were observed in 5 cases in patients with prior bone metastases in clinical remission and the remaining 3 cases in the absence of pre-existing bone metastases. The increased PAP and PSA levels, althouhgh present, showed less sensitivity in predicting disease progression related to bone metastasis.

**Table 1.** Increase of prostatic cancer marker levels before treatment

| | n | Osteo-calcin | PSA | PAP |
|---|---|---|---|---|
| With skeletal metastases | 27 | 22 | 24 | 23 |
| Without skeletal metastases | 25 | 0 | 21 | 19 |

**Table 2.** Prostatic cancer marker levels: response to hormone therapy (after 6 months)

| | Return to normal range | | |
|---|---|---|---|
| | osteocalcin | PSA | PAP |
| With skeletal metastases | 13/22 | 5/24 | 3/23 |
| Without skeletal metastases | – | 4/21 | 4/19 |

**Table 3.** Prostatic cancer marker levels: follow-up after 18 months

| Patients with progression of bone metastases | Increase | | |
|---|---|---|---|
| | osteocalcin | PSA | PAP |
| 8/52 | 8/8 | 6/8 | 5/8 |

## Discussion

Two cell populations are responsible for the continuous readjustement of the bone: osteoblasts with a fibroblastic origin and osteoclasts with a macrophagic origin. The former are responsible for osteogenesis, while the latter contribute to bone deconstruction [1]. The bone therefore maintains its equilibrium absorbing and releasing calcium, utilizing the balanced activity of these two cell populations.

To the present time, osteoblastic activity has been evaluated by measuring the alkaline phosphatase, an enzyme which is activated during the osteopoietic process, while the urinary hydroxyproline dosage must be obtained to evaluate the osteoclastic activity. This latter is an amino acid obtained from collagen degradation of the proteinic bone matrix. Neither of these markers are always specific and sensitive for evaluating the readjustment of the bone.

However, there are other proteins in the proteinic bone matrix that do not originate from collagen which have shown greater specificty. The vitamin K-dependent bone protein, osteocalcin, with a low molecular weight, is one of the most interesting of these. It is composed of 49 residual amino acids and has a marked capacity to bind to calcium [2].

The role of osteocalcin is that of regulating phosphocalcic homeostasis. It consistently increases when mineralization processes of the bone occur and it is therefore related to the hyperactivity of osteoblasts. Osteocalcin may be easily dosed in the blood with the radioimmunological method and, in our laboratories, 4–10 ng/ml values are considered normal in the adult male.

The correlation observed between osteocalcin increases and bone production processes has stimulated the curiosity of investigators in the search for always more reliable biological markers in the various bone diseases.

At first, knowing that this protein is exclusively bound to osteoblastic activity, attention was concentrated exclusively on evaluating and monitoring osteoblastic bone metastases. However, it was later observed that also in the presence of osteolytic bone metastases, tied to osteoclastic activity, the serum osteocalcin levels increased [3]. This apparent incongruity is justified by the understanding that a greater osteoblastic repairing activity, aimed at annulling the lytic effect of the osteoclasts, corresponds to every lytic bone activity. The osteocalcin level therefore follows this repairing attempt and increases its presence in the blood.

With regard to bone metastases in advanced prostatic cancer, osteoblastic metastases are involved in most cases and are thus related to an osteoblastic hyperactivity. This increased activity is usually revealed by higher osteocalcin levels in the blood. The mechanism with which bone metastases are formed in prostatic cancer appears to be related to a substance produced by tumor cells that stimulates osteoblastic activity [4].

Bearing these considerations in mind, the serum osteocalcin levels observed showed a great specificity for metastatic bone involvement. The PAP and the PSA levels, instead, did not behave in the same manner, as these are high even in the absence of bone metastases.

During hormone therapy in the bone remission. phase, osteocalcin levels tend to become normal, following its course with greater specificity than the PSA and the PAP. In addition, persistently high osteocalcin levels have, instead, been associated with a partial or completely absent response to hormone therapy.

Osteocalcin has proven to be extremely useful in follow-up as it has revealed, sometimes at an early stage, bone progression both in patients initially responsive to therapy as well as in those who did not present bone metastases at the beginning of the disease [5].

Osteocalcin is therefore useful to reveal bone progression, even during the course of therapy, presumably because of the appearance of hormone resistance.

The PAP and PSA values were useful to evaluate remission or disease development, with no particular correlation with the appearance of secondary bone lesions.

In conclusion, osteocalcin may play an important role in prostatic carcinoma as a specific marker of bone readjustement, useful both in the initial diagnosis and in monitoring during therapy.

## References


1 Owen M: Lineage of osteogenic cells and their relationship to the stromal system; in Bone and Mineral Research/3. Amsterdam, Elsevier, 1985, p 1.

2 Gallop PM, Lian JB, Hauschka PV: Carboxylated calcium binding proteins and vitamin K. N Engl J Med 1980;302:1460.

3 Francini G, Gonnelli S, Petrioli R: Is serum osteocalcin concentration a useful marker in patients with osteolytic osteoblastic and mixed bone metastases? J Tumor Marker Oncol 1988;3:321.

4 Francini G: Osteocalcina e metastasi ossee. Ligand Q 1988;7:340.

5 Francini G, Bigazzi S, Leone V, Gennari C: Serum osteocalcin concentration in patients with prostatic cancer. Am J Clin Oncol (CCT) 1988(suppl 2):583.

Eur Urol 1992;21(suppl 1):105–107

*C. Curatolo*[a]
*G.M. Ludovico*[a]
*M. Correale*[b]
*A. Pagliarulo*[a]
*I. Abbate*[b]
*E. Cirrillo Marucco*[a]
*A. Barletta*[b]

[a] Division of Urology, University of Bari (Dir.: Prof. *A. Piccinno*) and
[b] IRCCS (Dir.: Dr. *M. Di Lena*), Bari, Italy

# Advanced Prostate Cancer Follow-Up with Prostate-Specific Antigen, Prostatic Acid Phosphatase, Osteocalcin and Bone Isoenzyme of Alkaline Phosphatase

**Key Words**
Prostate cancer
Prostate-specific antigen
Prostatic acid phosphatase
Osteocalcin
Bone isoenzyme of alkaline phosphatase

**Abstract**
We report our experience in the follow-up of 63 patients with advanced prostate adenocarcinoma. We used prostate-specific antigen and prostatic acid phosphatase in 27 patients; in 36 patients we evaluated osteocalcin and bone isoenzyme of alkaline phosphatase, two markers of bone metabolism which seem to be good markers in the follow-up of patients with bone metastases.

## Introduction

Osteocalcin (OST) known as bone Gla protein (BGP), is a 5,800-dalton protein with a 49-amino acid structure, containing three γ-carboxyglutamic acid molecules. This protein shows affinity with hydroxyapatite; it is specifically synthesized by osteoblasts and is evaluated by RIA. Alkaline phosphatase is an enzyme produced during bone deposition. There are three of four AP isoenzymes. Rosalky and Ying Foo [1], Behr and Barnert [2] and Burlina et al. [3] describe a method to evaluate bone isoenzyme using a precipitation with lectin by wheat germ.

Many authors have studied prostate-specific antigen (PSA) and prostatic acid phosphatase (PAP) in monitoring prostate cancer. Sidall et al. [4] studied PSA and PAP in 51 patients with prostate carcinoma stage D2. 49 patients (92%) had PSA > 4 ng/ml, while only 35 patients (63%) had PAP values > 3.2 ng/ml. Oesterling et al. [5] evaluated PSA and PAP in 127 patients with prostate carcinoma before radical prostatectomy; in 64 patients (50%) PAP was > 3.2 ng/ml, while all patients had PSA values > 7.5 ng/ml. Stamey et al. [6] showed the correlation between PSA values and cancer progression during hormone therapy in 36 patients; they demonstrated that PSA is a good marker to identify a patient's response to therapy. Kuriyama [7] in 1,109 subjects showed PSA values > 2.5 ng/ml in 2% of patients without tested pathology, in 41% of patients with benign prostate hyperphasia and in 78% of patients with prostate cancer. In the latter group, PSA values were high in 69% of patients with stage A, in 70% of those with stage B or C, and in 82% of patients with stage D disease.

OST and bone isoenzyme of alkaline phosphatase (ISO-AP) are very new markers in the evaluation phase. Delmas [8] reported that 25 patients with primary hyperparathyroidism had OST values of about 14 ng/ml, while 29 patients with malignant hypercalcemia showed reduced values, and 18 with bone metastases had normal values. Lewenhaupt et al. [9] in 26 patients with advanced prostate cancer reported OST values > 5 ng/ml in 9 cases.

Dr. C. Curatolo
Division of Urology, University of Bari
Piazza G. Cesare-Policlinico
I-70100 Bari (Italy)


0302–2838/92/0215–0105
$2.75/0

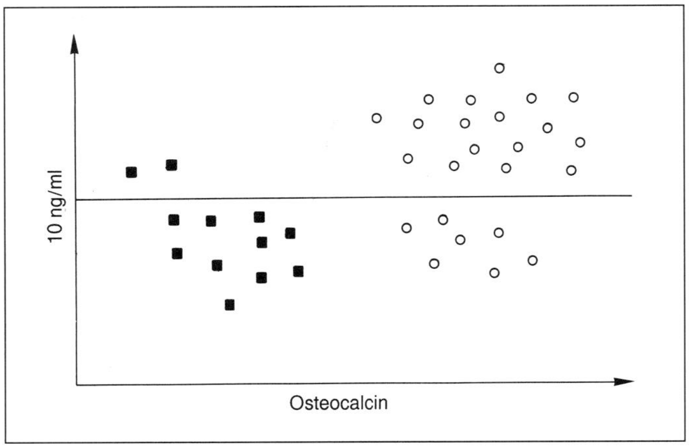


**Fig. 1.** Values of OST in patients with (○) or without (■) bone metastases.

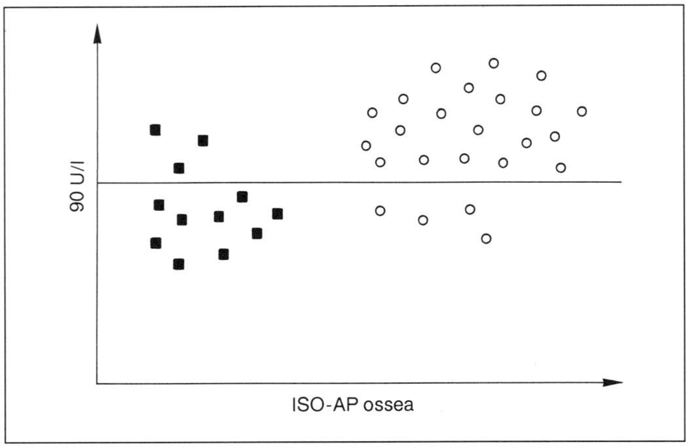


**Fig. 2.** Values of bone ISO-AP in patients with (○) or without (■) bone metastases.

**Table 1.** Evaluation before treatment of PSA and PAP in a group of 27 patients with prostate adenocarcinoma (18 with Gleason 3–5, 9 with Gleason 6–7)

| Treatment | | n | Gleason 3–5 | | Gleason 6–7 | |
|---|---|---|---|---|---|---|
| | | | n | % | n | % |
| PAP | < 3.2 ng/ml | 15 | 11 | 61 | 4 | 44 |
| | > 3.2 ng/ml | 12 | 7 | 39 | 5 | 56 |
| PSA | < 7.5 ng/ml | 4 | 1 | 5 | 3 | 34 |
| | > 7.5 ng/ml | 23 | 17 | 95 | 6 | 66 |

**Table 2.** Evaluation of PSA in 20 patients and of PAP in 9 patients after therapy with LHRH analogues and flutamide

| Treatment | | Patients | |
|---|---|---|---|
| | | n | % |
| PAP | < 3.2 ng/ml | 6 | 66 |
| | > 3.2 ng/ml | 3 | 34 |
| PSA | < 7.5 ng/ml | 18 | 90 |
| | > 7.5 ng/ml | 2 | 10 |

## Materials and Methods

Between January 1987 and January 1989, we evaluated PSA and PAP in 27 patients with prostate cancer stage D2, 18 patients had Gleason 3–5 while 9 had Gleason 6–7. These patients were treated with LHRH analogues and flutamide. Markers were tested before therapy and 6 months later with RIA. PAP cut-off was established at 3.2 ng/ml on a control group, while PSA cut-off was 7.5 ng/ml. Seric samples were practised 1 week after rectal examination or urethral manipulations. OST and bone ISO-AP were determined with RIA in 36 patients. Only 24 patients had bone metastases. The cut-off of ISO-AP was 90 U/l while in OST it was 10 ng/ml.

## Results

In the group of 27 patients, PSA was > 7.5 ng/ml in 23 cases (85%), while PAP was > 3.2 ng/ml in only 12 cases (44%) (table 1). After 6 months of therapy we evaluated PSA and PAP in the group of patients which presented increased values. 18 of 20 asymptomatic patients had PSA < 7.5 ng/ml, while 6 of 9 patients had PAP values < 3.2 ng/ml (table 2). In the group of 12 patients without bone metastases, OST was > 10 ng/ml in 2 cases (17%) while ISO-AP was > 90 U/l in 3 cases (25%). In the group of 24 patients with bone metastases, OST was > 10 ng/ml in 17 patients, while ISO-AP was increased in 20 cases (fig. 1, 2).

## Discussion

In advanced prostate cancer, bone markers such as OST and bone ISO-AP offer a new possibility in the evaluation of neoplastic progression together with PSA and PAP. In a group of 24 patients with prostate cancer stage D2, OST showed increased values (> 10 ng/ml) in 17 patients, while ISO-AP was increased (> 90 U/l) in 20 cases.

## References


1 Rosalk B, Ying Foo A: Two new methods for separating and quantifying bone and liver alkaline phosphatase isoenzymes in plasma. Clin Chem 1984;30:36–37.

2 Behr W, Barnert J: Quantification of bone alkaline phosphatase in serum by precipitation with wheat germ lectin. A simplified method and its clinical plausibility. Clin Chem 1986; 32:10–11.

3 Burlina A, Plebani M, Zaninotto M, De Nadai A: Gli isoenzimi della fosfatasi alcalina: metodi di determinazione e significato diagnostico. J Lab Med 1985;5:335–337.

4 Sidall JK, Cooper EH, Newling DWW, Robinson MR, Wealan P: An evaluation of the immunochemical measurement of prostatic acid phosphatase and prostatic specific antigen in carcinoma of the prostate. Eur Urol 1986;12: 123–124.

5 Oesterling JE, Chan DW, Epstein JI, Kimball AW: Prostate-specific antigen in the preoperative evaluation of localized prostatic cancer treated with radical prostatectomy. J Urol 1988;139:766–767.

6 Stamey TA, Kabalmin JN, Ferrari M, Yang N: Prostate-specific antigen in the diagnosis and treatment of adenocarcinoma of the prostate. J Urol 1989;141:1088–1090.

7 Kuriyama M: Prostatic specific antigen in prostate cancer. Int J Biol Markers 1986;2:67–76.

8 Delmas PD: serum bone gamma-carboxyglutamic acid containing protein in primary hyerparathyroidism and in malignant hypercalcemia. J Clin Invest 1986;5:77–78.

9 Lewenhaupt A, Elkman P, Enheroth P, Eriksson A, Nordstrom L: Serum levels of prostatic acid phosphatase, tissue polypeptide antigen, Ca-50, neopterin and of osteocalcin in patients with prostatic carcinoma. Scand J Clin Lab Invest 1985;45:330–334.

Eur Urol 1992;21(suppl 1):108–110

# Relationship between Prostatic Acid Phosphatase and Prostate-Specific Antigen Serum Levels and Prostatic Volume in Benign Prostate Hyperplasia

## Pitfall on Tumor Markers Assessment in Primary Prostatic Cancer?

*S. Omacini*[a]
*R. Mione*[b]
*M. Barichello*[a]
*U. Santucci Delli Ponti*[a]
*A. Bolgan*[a]
*G.P. Contemori*[a]
*S. Petracco*[a]
*G. Capitanio*[c]
*P.M. Donisi*[c]
*M. Gion*[b]

[a] Divisione di Urologia;
[b] Centro Regionale Specializzato per lo Studio degli Indicatori Biochimici di Tumore;
[c] Servizio di Anatomia Patologica, Ospedale Civile, Venezia, Italia

**Key Words**
Prostatic acid phosphatase
Prostate-specific antigen
Benign prostate hyperplasia

**Abstract**
Serum levels of prostatic acid phosphatase (PAP) and prostate-specific antigen (PSA) were measured in 78 patients with benign prostate hyperplasia and compared with both the gland weight and the glandular component of prostatic tissue. Both PAP and PSA were significantly higher where prostate was heavier; however, we could not find a consistent factor which could correlate weight increase to marker levels. PSA tended to be higher when glandular component was more expressed. From the present findings we conclude that in patients with prostate cancer, PAP and PSA serum levels should be investigated considering also the benign components of prostate gland.

Several investigators have identified a close relationship between prostate gland volume and both prostatic acid phosphatase (PAP) and prostate-specific antigen (PSA) serum levels in patients with benign prostate hyperplasia (BPH) [1–3]. Stamey et al. [4] demonstrated that an increase of 1 g of prostate tissue corresponds to an increase of 0.3 ng/ml of PSA serum level, although these findings have not been confirmed by other groups [5–8].

### Material and Methods

The present study was carried out between 1988 and 1990 and enrolled 78 patients who underwent subcapsular prostatectomy. Pathological findings were as follows: 44 cases (56%) with stromal glandular hyperplasia; 21 cases (27%) with BPH with complicated chronic phlogosis; 11 cases (14%) with BPH associated with various pathological findings (metaplasia, atypical hyperplasia, atrophy). Two patients (3%) with invasive adenocarcinoma foci were excluded from the study.

Preoperative serum samples for PAP and PSA assay were collected in basal condition or, in any case, several days (7–15) after eventual episode of acute urinary retention, endoscopic examination or digital rectal examination. The occurrence of acute or subacute symptomatic prostatitis was excluded. Patients were subdivided into three groups according to the prostate weight: (1) < 50 g (24 patients, 32%); (2) between 50 and 70 g (30 patients, 39%), and (3) > 70 g (22 patients, 29%).

Patients with not complicated BPH were further subdivided according to the glandular component which was histologically reviewed and related to the fibroleiomyomatous component. Four groups were arbitrarily identified with low (0–25%), intermediate (25–50%), high (50–75%) and very high (75–100%) percentage of glandular tissue.

Statistical analysis was carried out using the Mann-Whitney test and the Fisher exact test.

Dr. S. Omacini
Divisione di Urologia
Ospedali Civili Riuniti
I-30100 Venezia (Italy)


0302–2838/92/0215–0108
$2.75/0

**Table 1.** Relationship between PAP-PSA and gland mass in BPH

| Gland weight | PAP, ng/ml | | PSA, ng/ml | |
|---|---|---|---|---|
| | median | interquartile | median | interquartile |
| < 50 g | 1.9 | 1.5–2.5 | 3.5 | 2.7–4.3 |
| 50–70 g | 2.4 | 1.8–2.8 | 5.0 | 3.6–7.2 |
| > 70 g | 3.2 | 2.9–4.2 | 5.8 | 4.6–8.7 |
| | p = 0.0001 | | p = 0.0016 | |

**Table 2.** PAP and prostate weight: relationship with glandular component

| | Group A weight < 50 g gland. comp. < 50% | Group D weight > 50 g gland. comp. > 50% |
|---|---|---|
| Median | 2.85 | 3.80 |
| Interquartile | 1.85–3.15 | 2.55–4.95 |

Mann-Whitney test: p = 0.050.

**Table 3.** PSA and prostate weight: relationship with glandular component

| | Group A weight < 50 g gland. comp. < 50% | Group D weight > 50 g gland. comp. > 50% |
|---|---|---|
| Median | 3.85 | 6.20 |
| Interquartile | 2.75–6.28 | 4.10–8.80 |

Mann-Whitney test: p = 0.022.

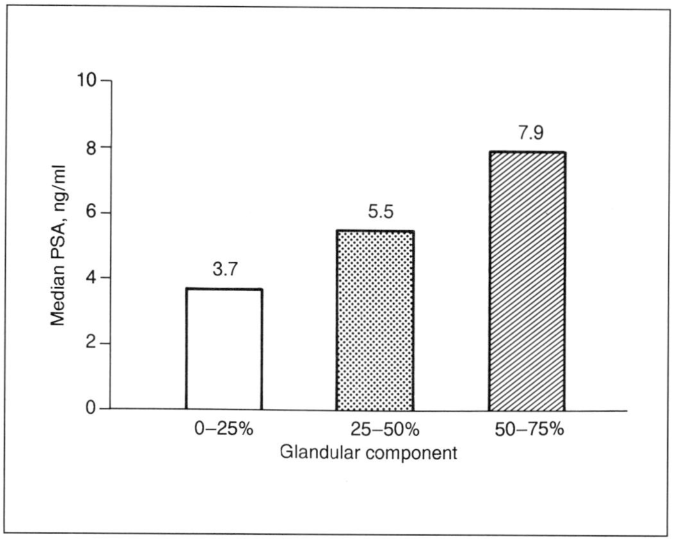


**Fig. 1.** Relationship between PSA and glandular component.

## Results

No statistically significant different PAP and PSA levels were found between simple and complicated BPH. Therefore, all patients were considered as a single group. A direct relationship was found between prostate weight and both PAP and PSA, with tumor marker levels being higher in heavier tumor (table 1).

When patients were subdivided only according to the percentage of glandular component, a not significant trend was found between the glandular component percentage and both PSA (fig. 1) and PAP (data not shown). Patients were further subdivided according to both prostate weight (PW) and glandular component (GC). The groups were as follows: group A: PW < 50 g, GC < 50%; group B: PW < 50 g, GC > 50%; group C: PW > 50 g, GC < 50%; group D: PW > 50 g, GC > 50%. PSA and PAP serum levels were significantly higher in group D than in group A (tables 2, 3).

The main drawback of several studies on the relationship between the weight of the prostate and other biochemical or clinical parameters is that gland weight was calculated on the basis of sonographic data. In the present study, only patients who underwent surgical prostate ablation were included. Therefore, prostate tissue has been actually weighted and no bias on this parameter should be expected. We could confirm a direct relationship between prostate weight and both PAP and PSA, the relationship being more evident for PSA. However, we could not demonstrate a linear relationship between the variation of weight and that of PSA, which was capable of giving a constant ratio between the increase of prostate weight and that of PSA serum level. Considering that PSA is secreted exclusively by glandular prostate tissue, we also evaluated the relationship between the marker and the percentage of glandular component in BPH. We demonstrated that PSA tends to increase with increasing percentage of glandular component, although without reaching the statistical significativity. However, it should be noted that subdivision of patients according to the glandular component was arbitrary and that the number of patients included in the study was not sufficient to evaluate the role of glandular component after stratification of cases according to prostate weight. When both prostate weight and glandular component were associated, it was possible to identify a group of patients with a gland weight $> 50$ g and a glandular component $> 50\%$ in which higher PSA serum levels should be expected.

From the present findings we conclude that, in patients with prostate cancer and a simultaneous BPH, serum levels of PAP and PSA should be evaluated taking into account both the weight and the glandular component of the benign prostate tissue.

## References


1 Ercole CJ, Lange PH, Mathisen M, Chiou RK, Reddy PK, Vessella RL: Prostate-specific antigen and prostatic acid phosphatase in the monitoring and staging of patients with prostatic cancer. J Urol 1987;138:1181.

2 Armitage TG, Cooper EH, Newling WW, Robinson MRG, Appleyard I: The value of the measurement of serum prostate-specific antigen in patients with benign prostatic hyperplasia and untreated prostate cancer. Br J Urol 1988;62:584.

3 Hudson MA, Bahnson RR, Catalona WJ: Clinical use of prostate-specific antigen in patients with prostate cancer. J Urol 1989;142:1011.

4 Stamey TA, Yang N, Hay AR, McNeal JE, Freiha FS, Redwine E: Prostate-specific antigen as a serum marker for adenocarcinoma of the prostate. N Engl J Med 1987;317:909.

5 Weber JP, Oesterling JE, Peters CA, Partin AW, Chan DW, Walsh PC: The influence of reversible androgen deprivation on serum prostate-specific antigen levels in men with benign prostatic hyperplasia. J Urol 1989;141:987.

6 Partin AW, Carter HB, Chan DW, Epstein JI, Oesterling JE, Rock RC, Weber JP, Walsh PC: Prostate-specific antigen in the staging of localized prostate cancer: influence of tumor differentiation, tumor volume and benign hyperplasia. J Urol 1990;143:747.

7 Barichello M, Gion M, Santucci Delli Ponti U, Bolgan A, Contemori GP, Cossaro E, Omacini S, Mione R, Bruscagnin G, Petracco S: Fosfatasi acida prostatica (PAP) e antigene prostatico specifico (PSA) in patologia prostatica. Impatto del metodo di dosaggio sull'informazione clinica. Acta Urol Ital 1991;V:1,51.

8 Wang MC, Papsidero LD, Kuriyama M, Valenzuela LA, Murphy GP, Chu TM: Prostate antigen: a new potential marker for prostatic cancer. Prostate 1981;2:89.

Eur Urol 1992;21(suppl 1):111–114

*Ü. Şimşek*
*S. Kutlu*
*İ. Yavaşçaouğlu*
*B. Oktay*
*M. Özyurt*

Department of Urology, Uludağ University, Bursa, Turkey

# Seasonal Variation of Prostatic Acid Phosphate and Prostate-Specific Antigen in Patients without Prostatic Malignancy

**Key Words**
Seasonal variation
Prostatic acid phosphatase
Prostate-specific antigen

**Abstract**
The seasonal pattern of prostatic acid phosphatase (PAP) and prostate specific antigen (PSA) in nonmalignant males was investigated. Serum levels were measured in 1,540 men during a 3-year period with radioimmunoassay methods using monoclonal antibody techniques. All of the tested individuals were free of prostatic malignancy. During each of the 3 years, PAP ans PSA showed a rise, especially in spring. The mean PSA level in spring showed a statistically important difference when compared with winter, fall and summer mean levels ($p < 0.05$). However, no significant difference of PAP levels was estimated seasonally in the 3 years, which shows that an important marker of prostatic cancer can vary with seasons.

## Introduction

The use of serum prostatic acid phosphatase (PAP) as a marker for prostatic cancers started more than 50 years ago [1]. Since then, its importance and characteristics have been studied extensively. The search for its diurnal pattern is a part of them. Over the course of the day its variance with the hours caused researchers to study its diurnal variation. The findings differ with each other but as a result, all of them agreed upon its variation but could not show a standard rhythm of it [2–5]. The other marker, prostate-specific antigen (PSA), is not so old as PAP. Since its discovery in 1979, many studies have been done on its various features. A few papers have been published on its diurnal pattern in prostatic and nonprostatic disease as well as in normal males [2, 6, 7]. The conclusions that the authors reached are similar to those of PAP. Having such a fluctuation in 24 h gave us an idea to search their monthly or seasonal pattern. With this study we tried to show one of their unknown characteristics.

## Materials and Methods

The aim of this study was to show the seasonal pattern of PAP and PSA in randomly chosen men without prostatic malignancy. For a period of 3 years (1988–1990) a total of 1,540 men were investigated for this purpose. Every month for 3 years, approximately 40 males were chosen and grouped. To equalize the groups, the number of males, their ages and diagnosed disease, we tried to equally disperse them. All of the blood samples were drawn in the morning hours and none of the individuals had undergone a rectal intervention like digital or ultrasonic examination 48 h prior to the test. An immunoradiometric assay (Coat-a-Count PAP, IRMA) was used for

Dr. Ümit Şimşek
Department of Urology
Uludağ University
Ducinar, Bursa (Turkey)


0302–2838/92/0215–0111
$2.75/0

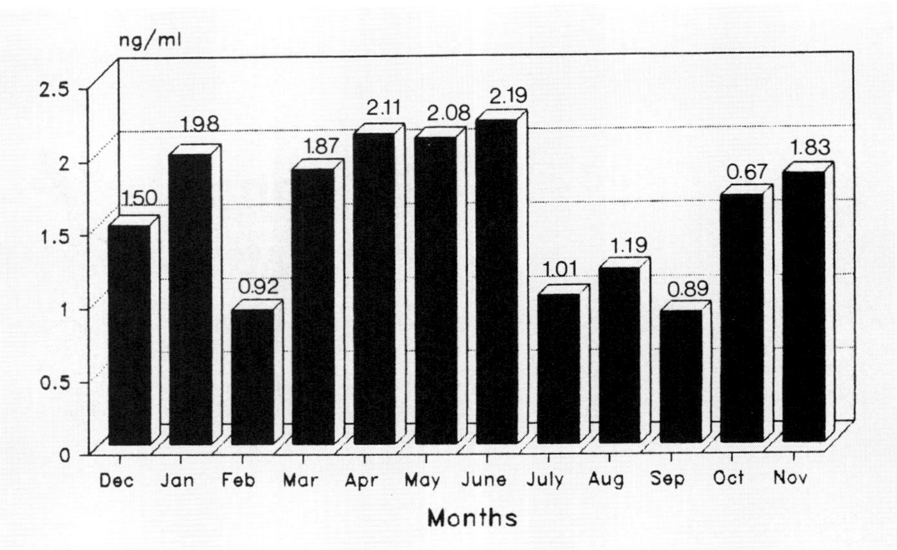


**Fig. 1.** Mean monthly levels of PAP in 3 years.

the determination of serum PAP levels. PSA was measured by the monoclonal anti-PSA antibody assay (IRMA-Count PSA). These techniques were used for the whole period of the study. According to the manufacturers, the normal value for PAP is 0–2 ng/ml and for PSA is 0–4 ng/ml. The mean levels of PAP and PSA for every month are calculated; they are then compared with each other using statistical analysis.

## Results

The ages of 1,540 men varied between 21 and 80 years (mean 35.1). In each of the 36 groups the mean age also varied from 34.6 to 37.1. The current status and the diagnosed diseases for the whole population are listed in table 1. We tried to use mostly the normal or voluntary males in our study so that the results would be more reliable. Therefore, more than half or the population was chosen from these individuals. The 'various other' group consisted mostly of urologic patients, but also of patients having tonsillitis, rhinitis, arthritis, bone fractures, lumbar disc hernia, peptic ulcus, gastritis, bronchitis, newly operated for acute appendicitis or inguinal hernia, etc.

Except for the BPH group, there was no or very little indication for the estimation of PAP or PSA in the population. Patients with prostatitis or prostatodynia were very small in number so that their effects would not have altered the results.

The mean levels of PAP are shown in figure 1 on a monthly basis and in figure 2 seasonally in the whole period of the study. From these two figures one can easily see the estimated high levels, especially in spring. June is another month that has the higher levels with is the beginning of summer. The difference between these seasonal PAP levels was not statistically important ($p < 0.05$).

In figures 3 and 4, the mean PSA levels according to the months and seasons are shown respectively. The highest levels are detected in March and April. The other spring month, May, did not show this striking raise but the seasonal mean level of spring was the highest of all other seasonal mean levels. The difference between spring and the other three seasons was statistically significant when compared one by one ($p < 0.05$).

**Table 1.** Distribution of diagnosis and current status of 1,540 men

| Current status/diagnosed disease | n | % |
|---|---|---|
| Normal (voluntary) | 840 | 54.5 |
| BPH | 320 | 21.0 |
| Prostatitis | 58 | 3.8 |
| Prostatodynia | 30 | 1.8 |
| Varicocele | 14 | 0.9 |
| Various other | 278 | 18.0 |
| Total | 1,540 | 100.0 |

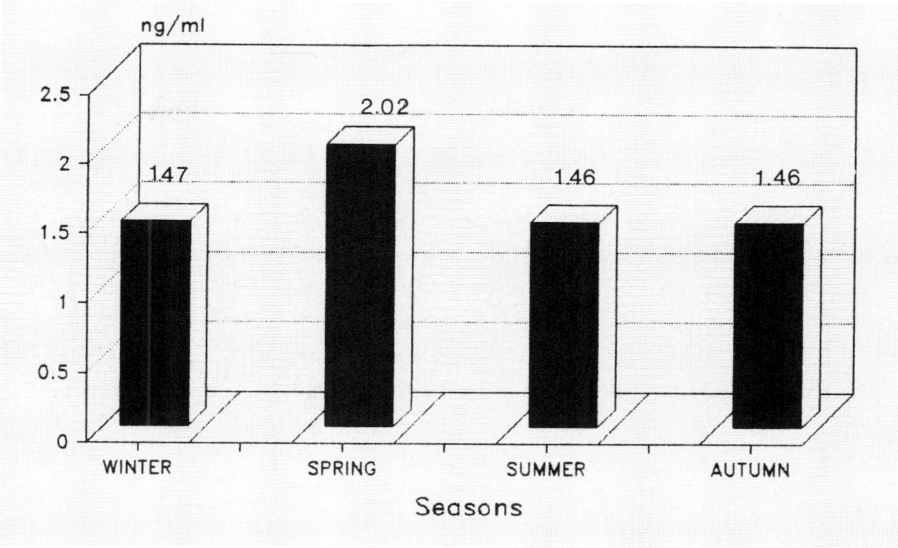


**Fig. 2.** Mean seasonal levels of PAP in 3 years.

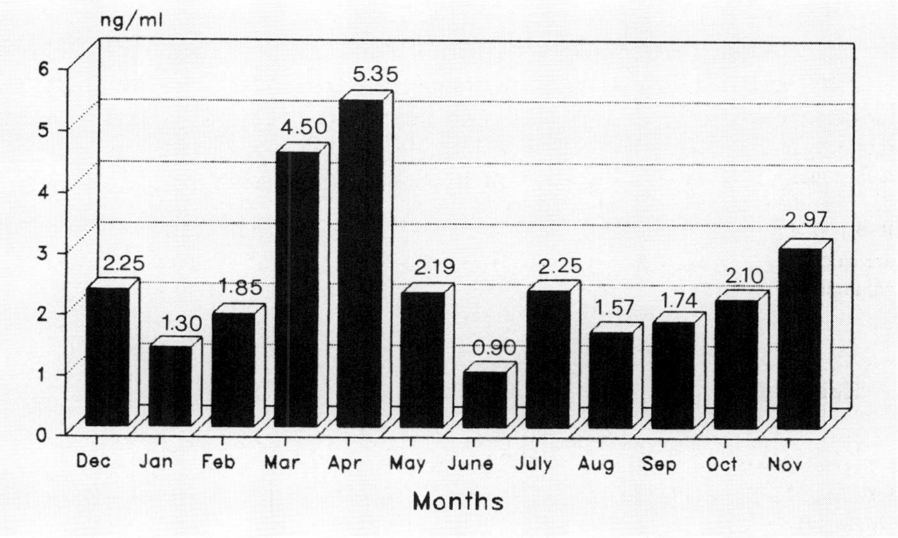


**Fig. 3.** Mean monthly levels of PSA in 3 years.

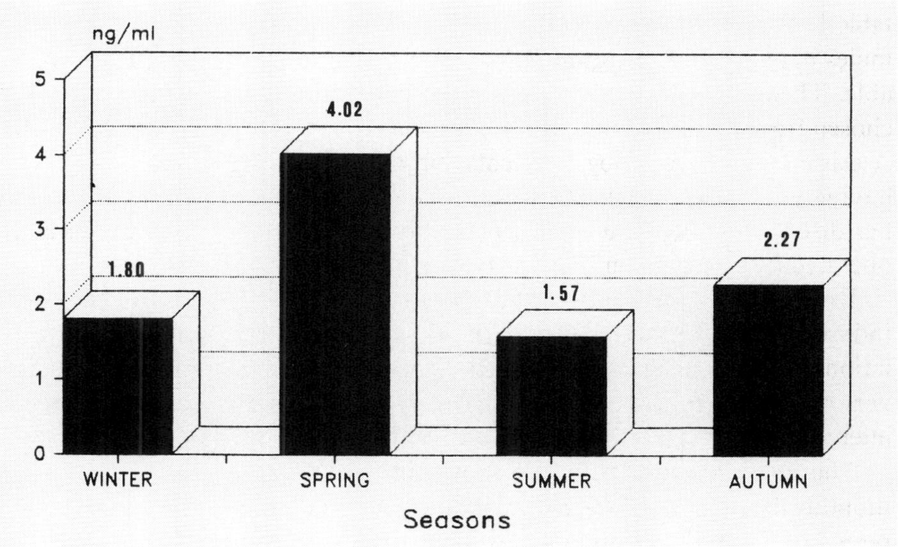


**Fig. 4.** Mean seasonal levels of PSA in 3 years.

## Discussion

At present, PAP and PSA are the only two, perhaps the most, reliable prostatic cancer markers. They are not 100% accurate. Many studies concerning their significance in some diseases other than prostatic carcinoma are also reported in the literature. Even in women, PSA is detectable in small amounts [8]. Being an enzyme or an antigen, they can easily be found in different tissues, or secreted by them, or can be produced in many conditions [7, 9]. These data bring out how easy we can measure false-positive levels of these two markers. They also fluctuate during the day. The papers that have been published on their diurnal pattern give different results [2, 4, 10].

As a conclusion we can say that both PAP and PSA do have daily fluctuations but they are so minor and unsteady that one cannot end up with a rhythm or a standard pattern. As far as we know, no study exists in the literature about their monthly or seasonal fluctuations. Human beings and the environment change a great deal with the seasons. We all very well know that there are certain clinical entities which increase in incidence with certain seasons. At present we do not have enough knowledge to explain the reasons. Peptic ulcus is a good example for this. PAP and PSA are also good candidates for this kind of behavior.

In our observation about PAP, we saw the little rises of its levels, especially in spring. This was not statistically significant, so we are not going to speculate on this finding. Perhaps some dilutional methods should be developed in order to get more accurate measurements. The same observation is also true for PSA levels. This time the rise detected in spring is much more prominent which was also found to be significant statistically. It is very hard to say something about this rise. We believe that these findings need to be supplemented with further studies and explanations. Spring time is the time of awakening for living things, that is, it is the time of increase of libido. This in turn can stimulate the glandular epithelium of the prostate where these two markers are secreted. The overproduction of these markers may also give rise to their blood levels which never exceed normal blood levels. The antigenicity of PSA is also a reason for its increase in spring.

The importance of the serial measurements of tumor markers is obvious, especially for the progression, regression or recurrence of the cancer. This observation is a good warning for the physician that a slightly higher level must be expected in spring for PAP and PSA.

## References


1 Henneberry MD, Engel G, Grayhack JT: Acid phosphatase. Urol Clin North Am 1979;3:629–641.
2 Dejter SW, Martin JS, McPherson RA, Lynch JH: Daily variability in human serum prostate-specific antigen and prostatic acid phosphatase: A comparative evaluation. Urology 1988; 4:288–292.
3 El-Shirbiny FMA, Pawar NH, Nilson GET: Diurnal variation of prostatic acid phosphatase in urologic patients with non-prostatic disease. Urology 1986;4:302–305.
4 Dejter SW, Erickson AB, Lynch JH: Characterization of secretion pattern of human prostatic acid phosphatase: A reassessment. Urology 1988;2:125–128.
5 Morse RM, Resnick MI: Detection of clinically occult prostate cancer. Urol Clin North Am 1990;3:567–574.
6 Wang MC, Valenzuela LA, Murphy GP: Purification of a human prostate-specific antigen. Invest Urol 1979;17:159–162.
7 Shearer RJ: Prostatic-specific antigen. Br J Urol 1991;67:1–5.
8 Morote J, Ruibal A, Palou J: Evaluation of specific antigen and prostatic acid phosphatase specificity. Study of false values. Int J Biol Markers 1986;1:141–146.
9 Brawer MK: Laboratory studies for the detection of carcinoma of the prostate. Urol Clin North Am 1990;4:759–768.
10 Nissenkorn I, Mickey DD, Miller DB, Soloway MS: Circadian and day-to-day variation of prostatic acid phosphatase. J Urol 1982;127: 1122–1124.

# Author Index

## Subject Index

# FLOBACIN®

(ofloxacin)

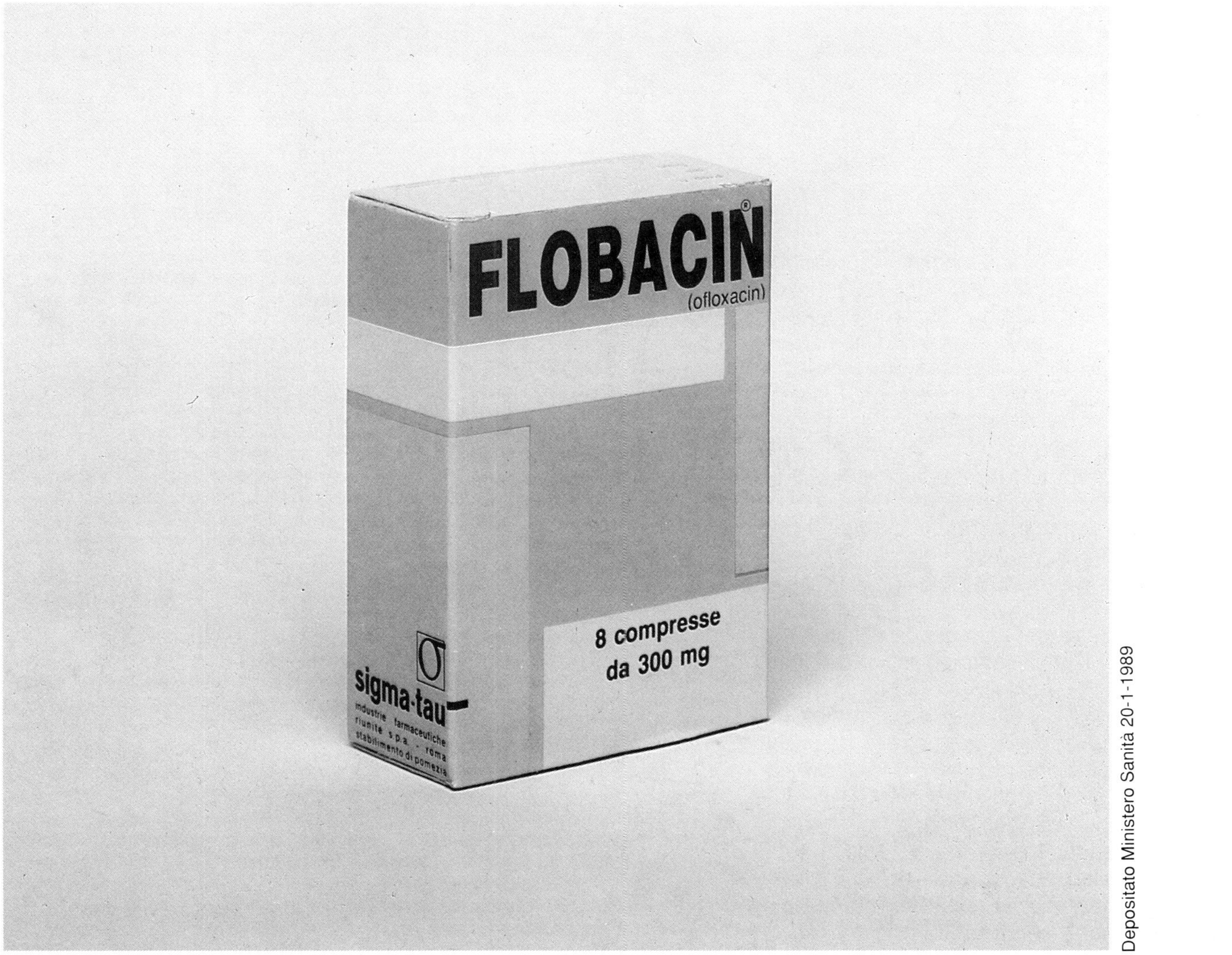


Depositato Ministero Sanità 20-1-1989

**CONFEZIONE:**
Astuccio da 8 compresse 300 mg

**sigma-tau** s. p. a.

prescrivibile
S.S.N.
Servizio Sanitario Nazionale

F 92054

**Progress in Experimental Tumor Research**
(ISSN 0079-6263), **Vol. 34**
Series Editor: G.A. Nagel, Zürich

**Editors: H. Eibl,**
**P. Hilgard, C. Unger**

# Alkylphosphocholines: New Drugs in Cancer Therapy

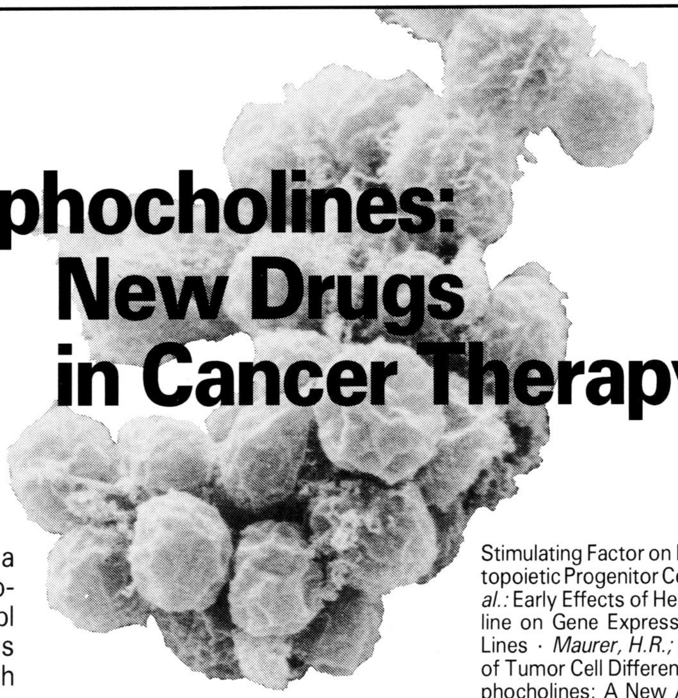

Alkylphosphocholines represent a new and exciting class of antineoplastic agents, discovered by Eibl and Unger, displaying numerous biological effects. The research presented in this volume focuses on the biological properties of hexadecylphosphocholine (HPC) – the prototype of this class and one of the first lipid-derived anticancer compounds to be brought from the experimental stage to clinical trial. The contributions, authored by scientists directly involved in these developments, discuss the selective antineoplastic activity of HPC both in vitro and in vivo as well as the application of HPC in the topical treatment of skin metastases resulting from breast cancer and lymphomas.
Summarizing what is now known about the biological activities of alkylphosphocholines and their potential as antitumor drugs, this book contains important new information for cancer researchers, oncologists and pharmacologists.

**Contents**



**Fields of Interest**

Oncology; Pharmacology, Pharmaceutics; Biochemistry, Cell Biology, Chemotherapy, Hematology, Immunology, Leukemia

Progress in Experimental Tumor Research, Vol. 34
**Alkylphosphocholines: New Drugs in Cancer Therapy**
Editors: Eibl, H.; Hilgard, P.; Unger, C. (Göttingen)
approx. X + 174 p., 85 fig., 32 tab., hard cover, 1992
SFr. 185.– / DM 222.– / £ 80.50 / US$ 148.00
US$ price for USA, £ price for UK only (subject to change)
ISBN 3-8055-5464-8

KARGER

KI92525

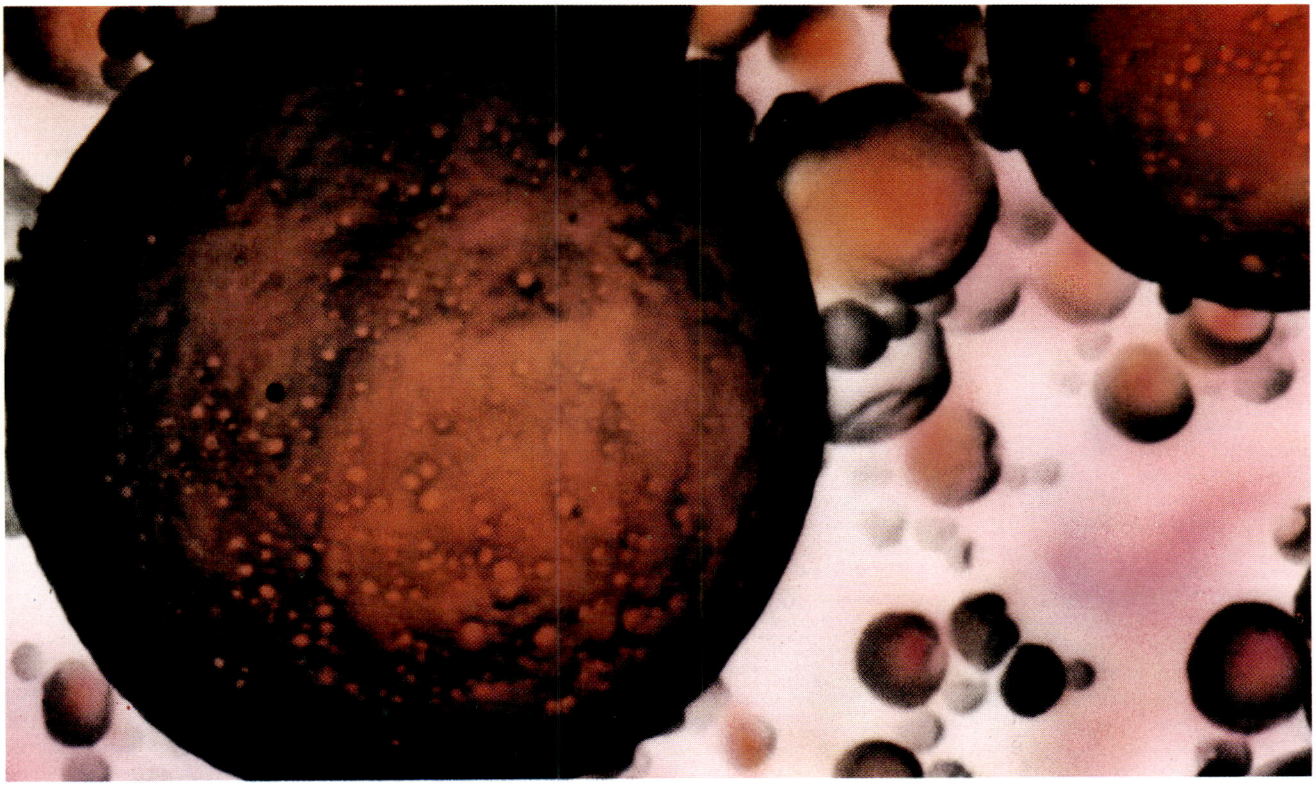

SCHEDA TECNICA ENANTONE DEPOT

**1. DENOMINAZIONE DELLA SPECIALITÀ MEDICINALE:** Enantone Depot.

**2. DENOMINAZIONE DEL PRINCIPO ATTIVO:** INN: Leuprorelin. USAN: leuprolide acetato.

**3. COMPOSIZIONE QUALITATIVA E QUANTITATIVA DEI PRINCIPI ATTIVI E DEGLI ECCIPIENTI:** 1 flacone di ENANTONE Depot contiene: **Principio attivo:** leuprolide acetato 3,75 mg. **Eccipienti**: Gelatina 0,7 mg, Copolimero di acido DL-Lattico e acido glicolico 33,1 mg, Mannitolo 6,6 mg. 1 fiala di veicolo per ENANTONE Depot contiene: Carbossimetilcellulosa sodica 10,0 mg, Mannitolo 100,0 mg, Polisorbato 80 2,0 mg, Acqua per preparazioni iniettabili q.b. a 2 ml.

**4. PROPRIETÀ FARMACOLOGICHE, TOSSICOLOGICHE ED ELEMENTI DI FARMACOCINETICA - 4.1. Proprietà farmacologiche:** Il leuprolide (INN: Leuprorelin) acetato, principio attivo dell'ENANTONE Depot è un analogo dell'ormone naturale LH-RH. Il leuprolide è molto più attivo dell'LH-RH naturale e può essere definito come superagonista del decapeptide fisiologico ipotalamico. Il leuprolide non è chimicamente correlato agli steroidi. L'ENANTONE Depot è formulato in modo da permettere, dopo la somministrazione, una continua ed uniforme liberazione del principio attivo dalla sede dell'iniezione, nell'arco di un mese. Dopo somministrazione di ENANTONE Depot si ha inizialmente un transitorio aumento degli steroidi sessuali per stimolazione della secrezione ipofisaria delle gonadotropine (effetto agonista). Entro 3 settimane dalla singola somministrazione si ha una inibizione secretoria dell'ipofisi (effetto antagonista) e soppressione della funzione gonadica. **Nell'uomo** questo produce una riduzione della testosteronemia ai valori caratteristici della castrazione che si mantiene per almeno 6 settimane. Con la somministrazione ripetuta ogni mese, la soppressione della testosteronemia si mantiene per tutta la durata del trattamento. **Nella donna** induce uno stato di ipoestrogenismo confrontabile con quello osservabile in menopausa. Con la somministrazione ripetuta ogni mese, questo stato di ipoestrogenismo si mantiene per tutta la durata del trattamento, causando una caduta dell'estradiolo e del progesterone, creando una condizione di "castrazione reversibile". Questi effetti possono essere utilmente impiegati in patologie ormono-dipendenti. Per quanto riguarda il carcinoma della mammella, oltre alla presenza di recettori specifici per il GnRH, è stata dimostrata una azione diretta degli analoghi dell'LH-RH sul tessuto tumorale indipendentemente dalla deplezione estrogenica. - **4.2. Proprietà tossicologiche:** La dose singola massima non letale nel topo e ratto per via parenterale è risultata essere maggiore di 100 mg/kg con il solo principio attivo. La $DL_{50}$ dell'ENANTONE Depot è maggiore di 2000 mg/kg per via i.m. Negli studi di tossicità cronica condotti su scimmia, ratto e topo non sono emersi effetti tossici inattesi ma solo effetti farmacodinamici ascrivibili al prodotto. Nel ratto trattato per 2 anni è emerso un trend (non statisticamente significativo) di adenoma ipofisario benigno. Queste modificazioni, che non trovano alcuna correlazione sull'uomo, sono ascrivibili alla specie animale impiegata ed alla farmacodinamica del prodotto. - **4.3. Farmacocinetica:** Subito dopo la somministrazione di Enantone Depot si verifica un picco ematico di leuprolide, cui fa seguito un livello di plateau proporzionale alla dose somministrata. Il prodotto viene rilasciato per circa un mese (4-6 settimane) in modo uniforme e costante (2,8%/die della dose somministrata) dal luogo di iniezione senza particolare differenza tra le vie di somministrazione (i.m., s.c.) e le 2 specie di animali impiegate (cane e ratto). In prove di somministrazioni ripetute non sono stati osservati fenomeni di accumulo. - **4.4. Cinetica ed effetti endocrinologici sull'uomo:** dopo iniezione di ENANTONE Depot si riscontra un incremento dose-dipendente delle concentrazioni sieriche di leuprolide. Entro 3 ore dalla somministrazione si raggiungono picchi sierici (fase iniziale di assorbimento rapido) a cui fa seguito la fase successiva di decremento o fase di lento rilascio del principio attivo che si protrae in modo costante per almeno 35 giorni dalla somministrazione. Livelli sierici di leuprolide sono ancora dosabili dopo 42 giorni. **Nell'uomo** la somministrazione unica di ENANTONE Depot ha prodotto (dopo un transitorio aumento entro la prima settimana) un rapido decremento entro 2-4 settimane dei livelli sierici del testosterone e del suo metabolita attivo, il diidrotestosterone, fino ai valori di castrazione in tutti i pazienti valutati. Tale fenomeno si è protratto fino all'ultimo periodo di osservazione dello studio (5ª-7ª settimana). **Nella donna** la somministrazione regolare di ENANTONE Depot comporta una soppressione della funzione gonadica che induce un'amenorrea ipogonadotropa.

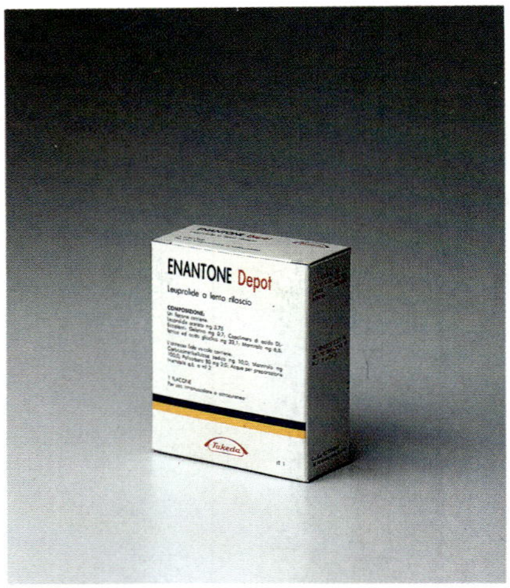


**5. INFORMAZIONI CLINICHE - 5.1. Indicazioni terapeutiche: Nell'uomo:** Ca. della prostata e suoi secondarismi. **Nella donna:** Endometriosi a localizzazione genitale ed extragenitale (stadi I-IV). Ca. mammario in donne in pre e perimenopausa ove sia indicato il trattamento ormonale. - **5.2. Controindicazioni:** Soggetti con accertata ipersensibilità specifica al prodotto. - **5.3. Effetti collaterali:** L'effetto più comune durante la terapia con leuprolide è rappresentato dalle vampate di calore secondarie alle modificazioni endocrine causate dal prodotto (soppressione della secrezione testosteronica nell'uomo e all'ipoestrogenismo similmenopausale nella donna). Altri effetti endocrini nell'uomo sono la diminuzione della libido, l'impotenza, la ginecomastia e la diminuzione del volume testicolare e nella donna diminuzione della libido, turbe mestruali, vaginiti con perdite ematiche. Altri effetti del farmaco nell'uomo sono rappresentati dall'iniziale peggioramento della sintomatologia ostruttiva urinaria (disuria, ematuria, dolore lombare), della sintomatologia muscolo scheletrica (dolori ossei) o dei segni neurologici da compressione (senso di debolezza o parestesie agli arti inferiori). Queste manifestazioni sono abitualmente transitorie e scompaiono in genere entro una o due settimane dall'inizio della terapia. Durante il trattamento con il farmaco sono stati inoltre segnalati i seguenti effetti collaterali: cefalea, nausea, vomito, turbe dell'alvo (stipsi o diarrea), anoressie, febbre, sudorazione, rash cutaneo, caduta dei capelli, vertigini, turbe del sonno (sonnolenza o insonnia), dolori generalizzati, parastesie, disturbi della vista, irritabilità, labilità emotiva, depressione, palpitazioni ed edemi periferici, dispnea. È possibile l'irritazione nel punto di iniezione. - **5.4. Speciali precauzioni per l'uso: Nell'uomo** l'inizio del trattamento è a volte accompagnato da accentuazione dei segni e dei sintomi clinici (in particolare dei dolori ossei). È stato segnalato, con gli analoghi dell'LH-RH, qualche caso di accentuazione di ematuria preesistente o di ostruzione urinaria, sensazione di debolezza o di parestesia agli arti inferiori. Queste manifestazioni sono abitualmente transitorie, scomparendo in una o due settimane dall'inizio del trattamento. Inoltre la possibilità di una temporanea esacerbazione dei sintomi durante le prime settimane di trattamento deve essere presa in considerazione nei pazienti con segni neurologici da compressione midollare o in quelli che presentano ostruzione urinaria. Può essere utile verificare periodicamente la testosteronemia che non deve essere superiore a 1 ng/ml. La risposta terapeutica può essere valutata a livello osseo attraverso esame scintigrafico e/o tomografico; a livello prostatico la risposta verrà valutata attraverso ecografia e/o tomografia (oltre l'esame clinico e l'esplorazione rettale). **Nella donna**, in caso di trattamento prolungato, può essere utile verificare periodicamente i valori di densitometria ossea in quanto gli analoghi LH-RH producono uno stato di ipoestrogenismo che induce una riduzione del contenuto minerale osseo. - **5.5 Impiego del farmaco durante la gravidanza e l'allattamento:** Sebbene non siano stati riscontrati effetti mutageni e teratogeni, il farmaco non va impiegato durante la gravidanza. - **5.6. Interazioni con altri farmaci:** Non sono state riportate interazioni con altri farmaci. - **5.7. Posologia e modalità di somministrazione:** Sia nell'uomo che nella donna il dosaggio necessario è pari a 3,75 mg (1 flacone) di principio attivo da somministrare una volta al mese. La durata del trattamento dell'endometriosi è di 6 mesi. Il contenuto della fiala veicolo va aggiunto al flacone contenente le microsfere liofilizzate. Il flacone così ricostituito va agitato onde ottenere una sospensione uniforme ed il contenuto, lattescente, va iniettato per via intramuscolare o sottocutanea. - **5.8. Surdosaggio:** In ricerche cliniche con il leuprolide acetato a pronto rilascio somministrato a dosaggi fino a 20 mg al dì e per la durata di 2 anni, non sono emersi effetti collaterali diversi da quelli osservati con il dosaggio giornaliero di 1 mg. In scimmie trattate per via s.c. e per 1 anno alla dose di 10 mg/kg/die non è emersa alcuna sintomatologia inattesa né alterazione dei parametri bioumorali non correlate con la farmacodinamica del prodotto. - **5.9. Avvertenze particolari: Nell'uomo** nella fase iniziale di trattamento con gli analoghi LH-RH, sono stati segnalati isolati casi di peggioramento della sintomatologia clinica, di tipo transitorio (vedi effetti collaterali). Ciò giustifica un controllo medico particolarmente attento durante le prime settimane di trattamento per i pazienti portatori di ostruzione delle vie urinarie e per i malati che presentano metastasi vertebrali. Per la stessa ragione, all'inizio del trattamento i soggetti che presentano segni premonitori di compressione midollare devono essere attentamente controllati. Nel periodo iniziale di trattamento, si può notare un aumento transitorio della fosfatasi acida. **Nella donna** affetta da endometriosi l'eventuale insorgenza di metrorragie gravi in corso di trattamento è da considerarsi anormale e comporta la verifica del tasso di estradiolo plasmatico che, se inferiore a 50 pg/ml, richiede indagini per l'identificazione di eventuali lesioni organiche associate. Tenere fuori dalla portata dei bambini. - **5.10. Effetti sulla capacità di guidare e sull'uso di macchine:** Non sono state segnalate interferenze.

**6. INFORMAZIONI FARMACEUTICHE - 6.1. Incompatibilità:** Non sono note incompatibilità. Il prodotto deve essere iniettato da solo - **6.2. Periodo di validità:** Il prodotto è valido per 24 mesi. - **6.3. Norme di conservazione:** Il farmaco può essere conservato a temperatura ambiente. - **6.4. Natura e composizione del contenitore primario. Confezione e prezzo:** Flacone di vetro di tipo 1, tappo in gomma butile, sigillo in alluminio. Confezione da 1 flacone 3,75 mg + fiala veicolo da 2 ml. Prezzo al pubblico L. 358.600. - **6.5. Ragione sociale e sede del detentore dell'autorizzazione alla immissione in commercio:** Takeda Italia Farmaceutici S.p.A. Catania - Officina di produzione Takeda Chemical Industries Ltd Osaka (Giappone) - su licenza Takeda Chemical Industries Ltd Osaka (Giappone). - **6.6. Numero di registrazione e data di prima commercializzazione:** Codice n° 027066012 Dicembre 1989. - **6.7. Eventuale tabella di appartenenza secondo la legge 22 dicembre 1975, N° 685:** Nessuna. - **6.8. Regime di dispensazione al pubblico:** Da vendersi soltanto dietro presentazione di ricetta medica.

Depositato presso il Ministero della Sanità il 16/10/1990 F 92058